Syncope

Editor

ROBERT SHELDON

CARDIOLOGY CLINICS

www.cardiology.theclinics.com

Consulting Editor

MICHAEL H. CRAWFORD

February 2013 • Volume 31 • Number 1

ELSEVIER

1600 John F. Kennedy Boulevard • Suite 1800 • Philadelphia, Pennsylvania, 19103-2899

http://www.theclinics.com

CARDIOLOGY CLINICS Volume 31, Number 1

February 2013 ISSN 0733-8651, ISBN-13: 978-1-4557-7069-4

Editor: Barbara Cohen-Kligerman
Developmental Editor: Teia Stone

Cardiology Clinics (ISSN 0733-8651) is published quarterly by Elsevier Inc., 360 Park Avenue South, New York, NY 10010-1710. Months of issue are February, May, August, and November. Business and Editorial Offices: 1600 John F. Kennedy Blvd., Ste. 1800, Philadelphia, PA 19103-2899. Customer Service Office: 3251 Riverport Lane, Maryland Heights, MO 63043. Periodicals postage paid at New York, NY and additional mailing offices. Subscription prices are $305.00 per year for US individuals, $508.00 per year for US institutions, $149.00 per year for US students and residents, $373.00 per year for Canadian individuals, $630.00 per year for Canadian institutions, $432.00 per year for international individuals, $630.00 per year for international institutions and $211.00 per year for Canadian and international students/residents. To receive student/resident rate, orders must be accompanied by name of affiliated institution, data of term, and the *signature* of program/residency coordinator on institution letterhead. Orders will be billed at individual rate until proof of status is received. Foreign air speed delivery is included in all *Clinics* subscription prices. All prices are subject to change without notice. **POSTMASTER:** Send address changes to *Cardiology Clinics*, Elsevier Health Sciences Division, Subscription Customer Service, 3251 Riverport Lane, Maryland Heights, MO 63043. **Customer Service: 1-800-654-2452 (U.S. and Canada); 314-447-8871 (outside U.S. and Canada). Fax: 314-447-8029. E-mail: journalscustomerservice-usa@ elsevier.com (for print support); journalsonlinesupport-usa@elsevier.com (for online support).**

Reprints. For copies of 100 or more, of articles in this publication, please contact the Commercial Reprints Department, Elsevier Inc., 360 Park Avenue South, New York, NY 10010-1710. Tel.: 212-633-3812; Fax: 212-462-1935; E-mail: reprints@elsevier.com.

Cardiology Clinics is also published in Spanish by McGraw-Hill Interamericana Editores S. A., P.O. Box 5-237, 06500, Mexico D. F., Mexico; in Portuguese by Reichmann and Alfonso Editores Rio de Janeiro, Brazil; and in Greek by Dimitrios P. Lagos, 8 Pondon Street, GR115-28 Ilissia, Greece.

Cardiology Clinics is covered in *MEDLINE/PubMed (Index Medicus)*, *Excerpta Medica*, *The Cumulative Index to Nursing and Allied Health Literature* (CINAHL).

Printed and bound by CPI Group (UK) Ltd, Croydon, CR0 4YY

Transferred to digital print 2012

Contributors

CONSULTING EDITOR

MICHAEL H. CRAWFORD, MD
Professor of Medicine, University of California,
San Francisco; Lucie Stern Chair in Cardiology
and Chief of Clinical Cardiology, University of
California, San Francisco Medical Center,
San Francisco, California

EDITOR

ROBERT SHELDON, MD, PhD
Professor of Cardiac Sciences, Medicine, and
Medical Genetics, Libin Cardiovascular
Institute of Alberta, University of Calgary,
Calgary, Alberta, Canada

AUTHORS

WAYNE O. ADKISSON, MD
Cardiovascular Division, Department of
Medicine, Cardiac Arrhythmia and Syncope
Center, University of Minnesota Medical
School, Minneapolis, Minnesota

LAURA ARBOUR, MD
Island Medical Program, Department of
Medical Genetics, University of British
Columbia, Victoria, British Columbia, Canada

LUCIANA V. ARMAGANIJAN, MD
Arrhythmia Service, Dante Pazzanese Institute
of Cardiology, Sao Paulo, Brazil

DAVID G. BENDITT, MD
Professor of Medicine, Cardiovascular
Division, Department of Medicine, Cardiac
Arrhythmia and Syncope Center, University of
Minnesota Medical School, Minneapolis,
Minnesota

DAVID J. BRADLEY, MD, PhD
Division of Cardiovascular Diseases,
Department of Internal Medicine, Mayo Clinic
College of Medicine, Rochester, Minnesota

SANTABHANU CHAKRABARTI, MD
Division of Cardiology, University of British
Columbia, Vancouver, British Columbia, Canada

GIORGIO COSTANTINO, MD
Unità Operativa di Medicina Interna II,
Dipartimento di Scienze Cliniche "L. Sacco,"
Ospedale L. Sacco, Università degli Studi di
Milano, Milano, Italy

JAUME FRANCISCO-PASCUAL, MD
Unitat Arrítmies, Hospital Universitari Vall
d'Hebrón, Universitat Autònoma de Barcelona,
Barcelona, Spain

RAFFAELLO FURLAN, MD
Unità Operativa di Clinica Medica, Humanitas
Clinical and Research Center, Università degli
Studi di Milano, Milano, Italy

JUAN C. GUZMAN, MD, MSc, FRCPC
Department of Medicine, McMaster University,
Hamilton, Ontario, Canada

**D.L. JARDINE, BSc, MBChB, DCH,
FRACP, MD**
Physician, Department of General Medicine,
Christchurch Hospital, Christchurch,
New Zealand

CLARENCE KHOO, MD
Division of Cardiology, University of British Columbia, Vancouver, British Columbia, Canada

ANDREW D. KRAHN, MD
Division of Cardiology, University of British Columbia, Vancouver, British Columbia, Canada

TRUDIE C.A. LOBBAN, MBE
Tylwych House, Newbold on Stour, Warwickshire, United Kingdom

CARLOS A. MORILLO, MD, FRCPC, FACC, FESC, FHRS
Department of Medicine, McMaster University; Director and Professor, Cardiology Division, Department of Medicine, Syncope and Autonomic Disorder Unit, David Braley CVSRI, Hamilton, Ontario, Canada

ANGEL MOYA, MD, PhD
Unitat Arrítmies, Hospital Universitari Vall d'Hebrón, Universitat Autónoma de Barcelona, Barcelona, Spain

VICTOR C. NWAZUE, MD
Research Fellow, Division of Clinical Pharmacology, Departments of Medicine and Pharmacology, Autonomic Dysfunction Center, Vanderbilt University School of Medicine, Nashville, Tennessee

JORDI PEREZ-RODÓN, MD
Unitat Arítmies, Hospital Universitari Vall d'Hebrón, Universitat Autònoma de Barcelona, Barcelona, Spain

SATISH R. RAJ, MD, MSCI
Assistant Professor, Division of Clinical Pharmacology, Departments of Medicine, and Pharmacology, Autonomic Dysfunction Center, Vanderbilt University School of Medicine, Nashville, Tennessee

NURIA RIVAS, MD
Unitat Arítmies Hospital Universitari Vall d'Hebrón, Universitat Autònoma de Barcelona, Barcelona, Spain

IVO ROCA-LUQUE, MD
Unitat Arítmies Hospital Universitari Vall d'Hebrón, Universitat Autònoma de Barcelona, Barcelona, Spain

COLETTE SEIFER, MB(Hons), FRCP
Director, Arrhythmia Service, Section of Cardiology, Department of Medicine, St Boniface Hospital; Associate Professor of Medicine, The University of Manitoba, Winnipeg, Manitoba, Canada

ROBERT SHELDON, MD, PhD
Professor of Cardiac Sciences, Medicine, and Medical Genetics, Libin Cardiovascular Institute of Alberta, University of Calgary, Calgary, Alberta, Canada

WIN-KUANG SHEN, MD
Division of Cardiovascular Diseases, Department of Internal Medicine, Mayo Clinic College of Medicine, Rochester, Minnesota

MARIA VIQAR-SYED, MBBS
Division of Cardiovascular Diseases, Department of Internal Medicine, Mayo Clinic College of Medicine, Rochester, Minnesota

Contents

> The most common form of syncope is reflex syncope (also called vasovagal syncope and reflex anoxic seizures). Reflex syncope is common, relatively simple to diagnose, and, in most cases, should not become a significant burden for patients or their families. Yet, too many patients with treatable syncope suffer dismissal of symptoms, misdiagnosis, and nondiagnosis at the hands of medical professionals. Clinicians can also focus on too narrow a range of potential causes for the symptoms. These factors can make the perspective of syncope and its care extremely burdensome, having a profoundly negative impact on patient well-being and quality of life.

> Syncope is a frequent cause for presentation to emergency departments and urgent-care clinics. The physician should establish a confident causal diagnosis, assess prognostic implications, and provide appropriate advice to prevent recurrences. An organized approach is needed to the assessment of the patient with syncope, including a careful initial examination as well as application of specialized syncope evaluation units and structured questionnaires for history taking. The initial patient evaluation, particularly a detailed medical history, is the key to identifying the most likely diagnosis. Based on these findings, subsequent diagnostic tests can be chosen to confirm the clinical suspicion.

> The overall risk for a patient entering the emergency department (ED) because of syncope ranges between 5% and 15%, and the mortality at 1 week is approximately 1%. The primary goal for the ED physician is thus to discriminate individuals at low risk, who can be safely discharged, from patients at high risk, who warrant a prompt hospitalization for monitoring and/or appropriate treatment. Different rules and risk scores have been proposed. More ad hoc studies are needed to define the prognostic and diagnostic roles of the brain natriuretic peptide and other noninvasive laboratory markers.

> Clinical decision making can be challenging regarding the emergency department (ED) management of patients with recent syncope. Several models of the syncope

putative pathophysiology of orthostatic hypotension, and suggests options for non-pharmacologic and pharmacologic management.

Most patients who present to a cardiologist with syncope have vasovagal (reflex) syncope. A busy syncope practice often also sees patients with postural tachycardia syndrome, often presenting with severe recurrent presyncope. Recognition of this syncope confounder might be difficult without adequate knowledge of their presentation, and this can adversely affect optimal management. Postural tachycardia syndrome can often be differentiated from vasovagal syncope by its hemodynamic pattern during tilt table test and differing clinical characteristics. This article reviews the presentation of postural tachycardia syndrome and its putative pathophysiology and presents an approach to nonpharmacologic and pharmacologic management.

Carotid sinus hypersensitivity was first reported more than 200 years ago. Nevertheless, a complete understanding of this relatively common clinical finding in older patients has proven elusive. There is evidence to support an association between symptoms, particularly syncope, and a hypersensitive response to carotid sinus massage. However, the clinical implication of a high prevalence in asymptomatic healthy older persons is not known. A central degenerative process likely underlies the pathophysiology, but this is as yet unproven. Although selected patients have had symptom improvement with treatment, particularly permanent pacing, there is a dearth of randomized controlled trial data to guide management.

Neurally mediated reflex syncope, more commonly known as vasovagal syncope (VVS), remains the most common cause of transient loss of consciousness and syncope in all age groups. Most evidence assessing treatment of VVS derived from randomized clinical trials is limited. Multiple modalities of both nonpharmacologic and pharmacologic strategies have been tested, with conflicting results. The treatment of VVS has been directed toward interventions that interrupt the reflex response at different levels, hypothetically preventing the onset of syncope. This article reviews the available evidence of the different nonpharmacologic and pharmacologic therapies available for the treatment of recurrent VVS.

The current evidence for pacemaker therapy is reviewed in 2 different syncopal conditions: reflex syncope with cardioinhibitory response and syncope in patients with bundle branch block. Although recent trials support the use of pacemaker therapy in selected patients with reflex syncope in whom an asystole is documented during spontaneous syncope or in whom an asystole is provoked with adenosine-5′-triphosphate administration, the best strategy in these patients and in those with syncope and bundle branch block is not well established. Ongoing clinical trials will answer this question.

The articles in this issue provide a comprehensive overview of the recent advances in the management of syncope by masters in the field. There are now solid approaches to most facets of diagnosis, risk stratification, prognostication, treatment, and health services delivery. However, 5 important challenges remain, including syncope etiology, treatment, health services delivery, and an individualized approach to syncope.

CARDIOLOGY CLINICS

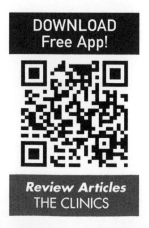

Foreword

CARDIOLOGY CLINICS

Foreword

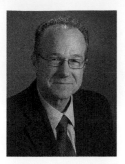

Michael H. Crawford, MD
Consulting Editor

Some might call syncope the low back pain of Cardiology. Data show that by age 75 the majority of people have had a least one episode. It is one of the top five nontraumatic reasons to visit an emergency department or urgent care center, and sometimes trauma is involved. In about half the cases we never find out why the patient fainted and have little clue about what to do for the patient. The differential diagnosis is enormous, ranging from cardiac to metabolic to neurologic to psychiatric causes. Someone once gave me a book that cataloged over 100 neurologic diseases that can cause syncope. Everyone's heard of Shy-Drager syndrome, but there were at least 50 more eponymic syndromes in this book. I wish I could remember the author's name, but unfortunately someone borrowed the book and never returned it.

Most cases of syncope turn out to be benign, but even garden-variety fainting can be disastrous if you hit your head. In some cases syncope is a harbinger of sudden death due to arrhythmias or mechanical obstructions in the circulation. It would be ideal to be able to separate these patients out for specific lifesaving therapy. In most states there are laws governing who can drive an automobile and who cannot after a syncopal episode. Reporting patients to the motor vehicle department is not a good way to

build your practice, but you may save the lives of some family in a minivan. Thus, evaluating syncope is complicated, serious business.

Last year at the American College of Cardiology annual meeting, I attended a symposium on syncope lead by Dr Sheldon and was astounded by the advances in the field and the clarity with which the speakers approached the challenges in this area. Thus, I was delighted when Dr Sheldon agreed to guest edit an issue of *Cardiology Clinics* on this important topic. Dr Sheldon has assembled some of the world's experts in syncope and provides his wisdom as someone who has devoted a large part of his career to this field. This issue will be of great value to clinicians who see these patients and researchers who hope to contribute to advancing our knowledge of syncope. However, be careful; someone may borrow this issue and never return it.

Michael H. Crawford, MD
University of California
San Francisco Medical Center
505 Parnassus Avenue, Box 0124
San Francisco, CA 94143-0124, USA

E-mail address:
crawfordm@medicine.ucsf.edu

Cardiol Clin 31 (2013) xi
http://dx.doi.org/10.1016/j.ccl.2012.11.001

Preface
Syncope—Now in Its Golden Era

After slumbering quietly for perhaps 3 millennia, the study of syncope entered its golden age about 25 years ago, with reports of the diagnostic utility of tilt testing appearing from Canada, the United States, and the United Kingdom. Although some debate has arisen about specific test methodology and the diagnostic accuracy of tilt testing, as well as its appropriate place in the diagnostic cascade, it is fair to say that it completely transformed the field. Before tilt testing, there was no diagnostic tool that was positive in high proportions of patients with syncope of unknown etiology, with reasonable specificity. We quickly learned that most of these patients had positive tilt tests, usually resulting in presyncope, syncope, hypotension, and inappropriate bradycardia. This provided investigators with a definable population of patients tied together by a history of syncope and by a positive diagnostic test. This in turn permitted studies of the physiology of vasovagal syncope, and large studies of its diagnosis, prognosis, and treatment, and health services delivery aimed at its care.

Now is a good time to synthesize and reflect on what we have learned. Trudie Lobban leads off this issue, describing syncope from the perspective of the patient, including her work in founding STARS. This was recognized by her receiving an MBE. Drs Adkisson and Benditt, whose 1989 article on tilt-table testing played a key formative role, provide a masterful overview of how and where patients present for care, and a general approach to their assessment.

Syncope assessment is proving to be extremely expensive and inefficient, and we are pleased to have 2 groups of experts from the United States and Italy describe recent advances in syncope assessment in the emergency department and in specialized syncope clinics. Following these, we review the 2 core diagnostic tools, tilt-table testing and implantable loop recorders. Khoo and colleagues provide a detailed and reassuring synopsis of identifying and assessing patients at high risk for arrhythmias, particularly young patients with rare genetic arrhythmias.

Before embarking on details of treatment, we turn to a thorough review of new advances in the physiology of vasovagal syncope. As David Jardine describes, the old notions of bradycardia and arteriolar dilation are now known to be only a small part of a rapidly emerging picture. Satish Raj and Colette Seifer describe several syndromes that frequently confound the diagnosis, including carotid sinus syncope, neurogenic hypotension, and postural orthostatic tachycardia syndrome. Finally, Guzman and colleagues take us through the evidence for medical therapy, and Moya and colleagues describe 2 fascinating advances in pacemaker therapy.

Altogether we are very fortunate to have so many talented clinical investigators provide these insights. I hope you will be as excited and fascinated while reading these articles as I have been.

Robert Sheldon, MD, PhD
Libin Cardiovascular Institute of Alberta
University of Calgary
3280 Hospital Drive NW
Calgary, Alberta T2N 4N1, Canada

E-mail address:
sheldon@ucalgary.ca

Cardiol Clin 31 (2013) xiii
http://dx.doi.org/10.1016/j.ccl.2012.10.011
0733-8651/13/$ – see front matter © 2013 Elsevier Inc. All rights reserved.

Syncope
A Patient and Family Perspective

Trudie C.A. Lobban, MBE

KEYWORDS

- Syncope • Misdiagnosis • Fainting • Blackouts • Patient • Family • Carer

KEY POINTS

- Accurate and timely diagnosis following transient loss of consciousness (T-LOC) is vital to identify potentially fatal underlying conditions and to prevent a dramatic reduction in the patient's quality of life.
- Accurate and timely diagnosis following T-LOC is frequently not achieved.
- Many patients endure a monodisciplinary approach to diagnosis that fails to explore all the potential causes of falls and T-LOC.
- Patients' symptoms are frequently ignored or dismissed as trivial.
- The impact of these factors on patients is significant yet commonly underestimated.
- The patient's perspective of syncope is often associated with burden, confusion, anxiety, fear, mistrust, and a significant deterioration in quality of life.
- Collaboration between appropriate clinical disciplines is essential for routine accurate diagnosis following T-LOC.
- STARS (www.stars-international.org) is a patient advocacy group for people with unexplained T-LOC. STARS works to promote collaboration, removing barriers to rapid diagnosis and effective management.

INTRODUCTION

The suffering of patients with syncope is frequently exacerbated by consultation with healthcare professionals.

Nearly 20 years ago, an advocacy group for patients with syncope was established in the United Kingdom (STARS, The Syncope Trust www.stars.org.uk). The defining characteristic of this group was its drive to encourage collaboration. Collaboration between different clinical disciplines and between patients and their clinicians and other professionals involved in the provision of care for patients with unexplained transient loss of consciousness (T-LOC).

In two decades, STARS has grown into an international nonprofit advocacy organization with an excellent track record of successful campaigning for better detection, diagnosis, and management of syncope. Throughout a host of lobbying victories, successful awareness campaigns, and award-winning educational initiatives; a single consistent theme emerges: collaboration eliminates barriers to change and results in improved patient care.

This article provides a tragic illustration of how the medical profession and its infrastructure can fail patients, but it also shows how collaborative efforts to drive change can lead to dramatic improvements in both the policy and practice of patient care. The author aims to show how engagement with the patient and a family perspective of syncope can reshape and save lives.

Founder and CEO of Syncope Trust And Reflex anoxic Seizures (STARS, www.stars-international.org), a global patient advocacy organization supporting patients who suffer from unexplained transient loss of consciousness.
Tylwych House, Stratford Road, Newbold on Stour, Warwickshire CV37 8TR, UK
E-mail address: trudie@stars.org.uk

Cardiol Clin 31 (2013) 1–8
http://dx.doi.org/10.1016/j.ccl.2012.10.004
0733-8651/13/$ – see front matter © 2013 Elsevier Inc. All rights reserved.

STARS

Imagine your son or daughter playing happily one minute and unconscious the next for no apparent reason. Your family doctor reassures you it is "something that can happen". Imagine it happening two weeks later; your concerns again being brushed off by your doctor, "stop worrying, no harm done." Worse, imagine your child losing consciousness up to eight times a day and still receiving no answers from clinicians, including those who witnessed your child blacking out.

Through determination and trust in a gut feeling that it is not normal for your child to faint, you begin a quest to find out what really is causing your child to lose consciousness whenever there is an unexpected pain, shock, or even a pleasant surprise. Countless letters to experts, numerous appointments and brain scans, yet no explanation is found. No answers despite hundreds of occasions when your little one is unconscious then sleeping for two to three hours to recover.

That was our life for more than 3 years before an arduous search led to a diagnosis. During that time, my daughter never left our sight for fear of injury during an attack. Through all this, my daughter's episodes came to resemble fits, her arms and legs jerking after she lost consciousness. In the absence of reassurance otherwise, we feared some form of epilepsy or perhaps even a brain tumor.

In desperation, we dispatched hundreds of letters to pediatric neurologists at children's hospitals around the world. Despite seeing consultants from some of the leading hospitals, we were left not knowing what could be wrong. Little did we know that hundreds, if not thousands, of others were enduring the same experience; appointment after appointment, test after test, only to be told nothing.

This is our story and the story of countless others who were also dismissed as simple fainters. Faint is often used to reassure patients that the problem is minor, and nothing to worry about. If you have ever fainted you will know that it is far from simple. When those faints are frequent and resemble fits, it feels alienating and insulting to be told they are nothing to worry about. And at no time before the eventual diagnosis was any mention made of a possible cardiac cause.

STARS was born from my terror, confusion, and frustration. Eventually my daughter was diagnosed with reflex anoxic seizures (RAS). I was told there was no treatment; however, the consultant pediatric neurologist who gave the diagnosis asked if I would consider speaking to other families in a similar situation. This began as an earnest effort to ensure that a niche group of parents would not have to endure the same fruitless and distressing

search for answers. It rapidly became something different. Following a brief appearance on a national breakfast TV show, the embryonic STARS was deluged with enquiries from thousands of parents and individuals who were experiencing, or had experienced, exactly the same battles for information, answers, and resolution.

STARS became a full-time job, rapidly growing from a kitchen table in a sleepy English village to an international network of offices, experts, and support teams all focused on the accurate diagnosis and management of T-LOC. STARS is now active in more than 30 countries around the world, addressing the common and unique challenges that prevent equitable and effective patient access to education, diagnosis, and management.

None of this progress would have been possible without the contribution of patients to clinical initiatives, or the contribution of clinicians to patient initiatives. STARS, from the beginning, had a Medical Advisory Committee (STARS MAC). This committee was the first of its kind in the world: a multidisciplinary group of clinicians from cardiologists to neurologists, pediatricians to geriatricians, even a psychiatrist. This layer of medical direction, insight, and credibility has been vital for the success of STARS, in the same way that an informed and confident patient voice has improved patient access to care via paths not readily accessible to clinicians or professional groups. Collaboration has routinely proved itself the best facilitator of progress.

Please visit www.stars.org.uk or www.stars-us.org for a wealth of educational information and practical tools for both patients and clinicians.

T-LOC and Syncope

Nontraumatic episodes of T-LOC caused by a reduction of blood flow to the brain are called syncope.[1–3] Syncope is the most frequent cause of T-LOC,[4] and it affects a great many people in westernized populations; its lifetime risk is estimated at 39% and it affects women (47%) roughly twice as frequently as men (24%).[5] Syncope can be an indication of a potentially fatal underlying arrhythmia.[6] Other causes, if undiagnosed or inadequately managed, can result in a significant reduction in quality of life.[7] Consequently, it becomes vital that diagnosis is reached rapidly and accurately in patients presenting with T-LOC.

Syncope is relatively simple to diagnose and can be managed adequately in many cases.[8] It has been shown that a good rate and accuracy of diagnosis can be achieved in clinical practice. With just a comprehensive medical history, a physical examination, and an electrocardiograph (ECG), 63% of patients can be diagnosed. The diagnostic accuracy associated with this rate was found to be 91%.[8]

THE CHALLENGE OF DIAGNOSIS

These findings are often reported in a manner suggesting that syncope is routinely and accurately diagnosed and that, if all physicians took a suitably comprehensive history, conducted an adequate physical examination with an ECG; then the problem of undiagnosed and misdiagnosed syncope would be eliminated. First, this implication might incautiously overlook the 37% of patients for whom initial investigations prove inconclusive. Second, it also risks trivializing the scale of the task required to implement effective initial consultations with patients with T-LOC within time and resource restrictions.

The prevailing clinical evidence illustrates the extent to which the diagnostic ideal is not achieved; in 1 study, 50% of patients with T-LOC were discharged from hospital with no diagnosis.[9] In several studies focusing on the misdiagnosis of epilepsy, it has consistently been found that around 40% of patients with epilepsy are misdiagnosed[10–12] and around 60% of these have been found to have syncope.[10] This highlights not just the routine difficulties of diagnosing syncope but the need to ensure that the onward path of patients initially undiagnosed engages a multidisciplinary healthcare team that maintains a sufficiently broad perspective on the possible causes of the presenting symptoms.

Among those patients for whom an immediate accurate diagnosis is not possible, and for those not fortunate enough to benefit from a sufficiently thorough assessment, the outlook can be bleak (**Box 1**).

Box 1
The challenge of diagnosis

- Syncope should not be burdensome for patients.
- Reflex syncope has a lifetime risk of 39%.
- More than 60% of syncope cases should be accurately diagnosed at first consultation.
- Misdiagnosis and nondiagnosis are common.
- Syncope is avoidably burdensome for a significant minority of patients.
- Many of these patients only learn of syncope after many years, if ever, after desperate searching and suffering.

THE PATIENT PERSPECTIVE

The patient perspective of syncope is dependent on several factors. For many, however, the most important influence is often the quality of information they receive on initial presentation, particularly with regard to possible diagnoses and on routes to securing a diagnosis. After an initial consultation, a patient should feel reassured, supported, empowered, and on a path to resolution, even when an accurate diagnosis is not achieved. Consistent with the evidence already reviewed, direct accounts from patients demonstrate that consultations with clinicians frequently result in outcomes far distant from this ideal. Not only is the opportunity for routine diagnosis missed, steps follow that further compromise and delay the diagnostic process. The patient then becomes disempowered, confused, anxious, and unsupported, sometimes for many years. In extreme cases, the resulting impact on well-being and quality of life is both tragic and enduring.

As a patient advocacy organization, we usually only hear from patients sufficiently deep into a fruitless search to have become frustrated to the point of desperation and anger. Despite being routinely surprised by the unique circumstances and events described, we commonly encounter two primary obstacles to the effective diagnosis and treatment of syncope patients. Failure to navigate these obstacles burdens patients and their families with considerable anxiety while symptoms continue to affect quality of life. Moreover, misdiagnosis can result in inappropriate treatments and iatrogenic effects that further burden patients, robbing them of their freedom, health, and peace of mind. The two obstacles to effective diagnosis and management of syncope that are most commonly encountered are:

1. Dismissal of trivial symptoms
2. Misdiagnosis following a narrow focus on possible cause, usually:
   a. Falls
   b. Seizures

NONDIAGNOSIS FOLLOWING DISMISSAL OF SYMPTOMS

In practice, these obstacles commonly occur together. The following case study provides insight into just how prevalent and damaging the dismissal of symptoms can be.

Case Study 1: James, Symptoms Dismissed

James, a 45-year-old man, was 13 years old when he first suffered T-LOC. The professional advice received amounted to "it's just one of those things". James and his family were advised that there was nothing to be done but learn to live with it. For more than 20 years, they did. As experience of the episodes grew, they learned to identify triggers. After two decades they had a long list, including loud bangs, pain, illness, and alcohol. As the list grew, so did the length of the unconscious spells and the duration needed for recovery.

Aged 35 years, James had a particularly dramatic T-LOC while on vacation. A physician who provided assistance at the scene recommended that the family seek a referral to check for syncope once they returned home. This was the first time a medical professional had provided mention of a diagnosis, let alone the potential for successful treatment. This information led to a dramatic increase in confidence that the family might be able to find help to prevent the episodes.

Back home, a neurologist, unable to stimulate an episode on a tilt table, decided against syncope and advised only avoidance of triggers. Avoiding triggers at this point ruled out much that constitutes a normal life. Three years later, James was admitted to the emergency department with a suspected cardiac arrest. On regaining consciousness, James explained his history, received further inconclusive tilt-table tests and, once again, was sent home with no diagnosis, just advice to live with it as best he could. Determined to understand more, James' own research led him to STARS, which was able to direct him to a specialist unit. During the first visit to this unit, the team diagnosed reflex syncope with asystole and scheduled pacemaker implantation. James has suffered no further attacks and is living a normal life for the first time in more than 20 years.

This account is not particularly unusual. STARS has many examples on file that illustrate lengthy and convoluted routes to diagnosis and treatment experienced by patients throughout the world. What is unusual in this account is the dispassionate way in which it has been presented. Little of the family's angst, despair, or anxiety is touched on. The restrictions that gradually applied to James and his wife's lives are largely omitted, as are the many severe injuries and inconveniences James suffered as a result of his regular falls.

This case highlights the importance of a thorough history and careful adherence to a structured diagnostic process. James and his wife estimate that they sought information, diagnosis, and treatment for the episodes from more than 30 physicians. Of these, only two provided guidance and medical assistance that led to diagnosis and effective management. In many ways James was unlucky, repeatedly being dismissed by expert physicians,

even after he and his wife had become aware that syncope might be the cause. Regardless of this poor fortune, the case illustrates a general lack of awareness of syncope and a swiftness to disregard symptoms instead of pursuing a comprehensive diagnostic path.

Awareness of the patient's perspective of their condition also needs to inform the language and approach used when providing vital reassurance. A patient who has suffered months or years of dismissal, unexplained T-LOC, fear, and anxiety is unlikely to respond well to being heartily advised that the problem is just a simple faint (**Box 2**).

MISDIAGNOSIS AFTER A SEIZURE

From case studies collected over several years, it became apparent to the Medical Advisory Committee of STARS that many patients were starting a long and often frustrating journey after an initial referral to a neurologist with suspected epilepsy. Such a referral is understandable given the myoclonic jerks experienced by many patients with reflex syncope during an episode. It was also common that, after failure to control seizures with antiepileptic medication, little further investigation of cause took place until the patient initiated a discussion on syncope or demanded another opinion.

Evidence of misdiagnosis among patients with epilepsy demonstrates that these observations might be the foundation of a general effect (**Box 3**). As has already been noted, the rate of misdiagnosis for epilepsy is high. Data suggest that up to 40% of adults and children with an epilepsy diagnosis are misdiagnosed, and that 60% of these actually have reflex syncope.[10–12]

Because syncope is most common in the young and the elderly, STARS encounters many cases of reflex syncope in teenagers and young adults misdiagnosed as epilepsy. A common feature of these

---

Box 2
Dismissal of patient symptoms

- The power of reassurance "that it's nothing" should not be overestimated. Lives can be blighted for years through a desire not to trouble the doctor.

- Tests for syncope, like epilepsy, are far from straightforward. A negative tilt-table test does not constitute evidence of nonsyncope.

- Incomplete investigation of the cause of faints, falls, blackouts, and seizures can easily lead to the dismissal of trivial symptoms that can result in debilitating or fatal consequences.

Box 3
Misdiagnosis after a seizure

Box 3
Misdiagnosis after a seizure

- There is considerable evidence that syncope is frequently misdiagnosed as epilepsy.
- Syncope is not a condition exclusive to the young or the old.
- Syncope has a strong genetic component. Exploration for similar incidents among family members is encouraged.
- The long-term consequences of misdiagnosis can be extremely burdensome.

case studies is that, after referral to an epilepsy specialist, other potential causes are no longer considered.

Case study 2 highlights the tragedy that can be inflicted on a patient when a single line of diagnostic enquiry is followed too narrowly.

Case Study 2: Angeline, Misdiagnosed with Epilepsy

Angeline first experienced faints at the age of 6 years, ranging in frequency from 5 to 15 times a year and often associated with emotional stress. The family doctor referred her to a cardiologist with concern about an errant heartbeat. They were sent home by the specialist assured that it was something that she would grow out of. Angeline was prescribed diazepam for her mother to administer in stressful situations. Aged 10 years, the faints became more like fits, resulting in referral to a neurologist who diagnosed epilepsy. The diagnosis revolutionized her life for the worse. She was excluded from many school activities. She was no longer invited to friends' parties. She was not even allowed to lock the bathroom door. This loss of privacy and social engagement became considerably more burdensome as Angeline moved into her teens. The antiepilepsy medication failed to control her so-called seizures but burdened her with a host of side effects.

In her early 20s, Angeline had a daughter who had an episode of T-LOC at the age of 2 years. Fears of epilepsy were allayed during consultation with a pediatrician who diagnosed RAS, which, they were advised, required no treatment and would pass with time. Repeated consultations to help reduce the impact of both her own and her daughter's attacks resulted in no more than general reassurance.

At age 30 years, Angeline's attacks worsened, as had her daughter's RAS. Angeline's husband began to notice similarities between the attacks his wife and daughter experienced. Pursuing the possible implications of these similarities, the family contacted STARS who directed them to an electrophysiologist with an interest in syncope.

At age 39 years, Angeline was told that she did not have epilepsy and was diagnosed with vasovagal syncope. After advice and treatment with a pacemaker, Angeline suffered no further T-LOC and has since been discovering how to lead a normal life, angry at all the anxiety and depression she needlessly endured, along with all the freedoms she and her family did without.

Her eldest daughter, who also fainted, has since received a pacemaker after episodes of asystole of up to 45 seconds were recorded. Her father was told he suffered with a virus for 9 years after several episodes of fainting; he too has now been correctly diagnosed and treated after contact with STARS.

The whole family had been blighted for almost 30 years due to misdiagnosis, inappropriate drug treatment to the point when the husband gave up his career in the armed forces to move closer to Angeline's parents. She could not be left alone with young children in case she blacked out and not only injured herself but also their children.

Angeline applied for jobs but always had to produce documentation to prove she was fit to work. Since being correctly diagnosed and treated, she is able to lead an active, productive life.

NONDIAGNOSIS AFTER A FALL

The age distribution of syncope has two peaks. The first is in children and young adults, predominantly in females. The second peak occurs with more elderly patients. Among these patients, the danger of falls is well recognized and the prevention of falls is a well-developed sphere of activity and research. Less recognized is the potential for syncope to be the root cause of falls in this population.

The following case study illustrates the personal and professional impact of falls that are not sufficiently broadly investigated (**Box 4**).

Case Study 3: June, Lack of Diagnosis After a Fall

Aged 56 years, June had a high-pressure, high-profile job. That year she also began suffering

Box 4
Nondiagnosis after a fall

- The value of a multidisciplinary approach is compromised if appropriate expertise is not sought.
- Knowledge of T-LOC and its possible causes among nonelectrophysiologists remains low.

from unexplained falls once every two weeks. At work, it was joked that she drank too much or the heels on her shoes were too high. After several months of regular falls, she sought medical advice. Within weeks, she underwent magnetic resonance imaging (MRI) and a computed tomography (CT) scan, and her falls were investigated by several neurologists, an ophthalmologist, a rheumatologist, and an ear, nose, and throat consultant. Many conditions were tested for and ruled out. One clinician prescribed β-blockers but these exacerbated the problem. Not only was this gamut of medical investigations fruitless, June had begun to feel that the clinicians she consulted thought she was neurotic; making a fuss about nothing.

Three years later, June eventually lost her job as she could no longer perform to a high level of commitment because of the number of falls, subsequent injury, and time away from work. After contacting STARS following an Internet search, June again sought medical advice, this time from her husband's physician who, after taking a comprehensive history, reviewed June's medical records and referred the case to a cardiologist with suspected syncope. The specialist shared the suspicion and implanted a loop recorder to confirm. Five years after the first instance of T-LOC, June received a pacemaker; her falls stopped, allowing her to return to a life she had all but abandoned.

ENCOURAGING AN APPROPRIATE MULTIDISCIPLINARY APPROACH

As noted earlier and highlighted in the case studies, diagnosis of patients with T-LOC benefits from a multidisciplinary approach. T-LOC most commonly results from epilepsy, syncope, and psychogenic causes. In addition, many patients are admitted due to a fall that was precipitated by syncope, a detail that often goes uninvestigated and unrecognized.

The addition of a patient voice proved invaluable in the development of services to address these needs. STARS, with guidance from its Medical Advisory Committee, began advocating the need for research and development of clinics specifically for the referral of patients presenting with unexplained T-LOC. Rapid Access T-LOC Clinics (RATCs) were the result of this effort. RATCs are notable for their reliance on input from multiple relevant disciplines (neurology, cardiology, and gerontology), the use of a standard and comprehensive patient questionnaire to ensure a thorough and pertinent history, and the review of cases in light of all possible causes before a diagnostic and treatment approach is agreed. These clinics are pointedly not called Syncope Clinics. By labeling these clinics T-LOC (or Blackout, according to the prevailing culture), no presupposition of a diagnosis is inherent in the referral, encouraging the referral of patients that might not be sent to a syncope or a falls clinic. The diagnostic pathway remains as open as possible.

Several RATCs have been established in the United Kingdom, delivering considerable success notably in Manchester, Middlesborough, and Wolverhampton. Current efforts are promoting the establishment of additional clinics throughout the regions of the United Kingdom and around the world.

In 2013, STARS will launch the Rapid Access T-LOC Web site. This site will contain all the guidance and resources necessary to establish an RATC, including clinical data on their success and access to a standard online patient questionnaire and data aggregation service. The service will go live at www.starstloc.org.

EQUIPPING AND EMPOWERING PATIENTS

Patient advocacy groups take many forms but they invariably become established in response to gaps in the healthcare system to fulfill a need that is often underappreciated by medical professionals but has a profoundly negative impact on the lives of patients and their carergiver's seeking answers and direction. In an ideal healthcare system, patient advocacy groups would not exist. That they do, and that they are so vocal and influential, is frequently illustrative of the depth of need that is not being addressed.

STARS seeks to create and redesign effective health care services, and works to improve the plight of T-LOC patients through educational tools and materials. The most successful and widely distributed item of patient literature ever developed by STARS was specifically designed to maximize the likelihood of collaborative and open discussion on the causes of T-LOC between healthcare professionals and patients. The Blackouts Checklist (or T-LOC or Fainting Checklist, depending on the prevailing preference) was designed to educate, equip, and motivate a patient for consultation with general and specialist physicians on unexplained T-LOC. The Checklist then became a highly effective piece of educational literature for healthcare professionals.

The Checklist provides an excellent example of how patient and physician education can be advanced through the constructive and focused collaboration of clinical experts and patient groups. A reprint of the current UK version of the Checklist is given in the following page. For further reference, the current UK checklist is available

<table>
<tr><td>

Box 5
Topics addressed by the Blackouts Checklist Information Booklet

- Why people experience spells of unconsciousness
- Common diagnostic challenges
- Preparing for a doctor's appointment
- Preparing patient and witness accounts of blackouts
- The need for multiple experts to work together
- What to expect in hospital
- Questions to prepare for
- Questions to ask

</td></tr>
</table>

online at www.stars.org.uk/patient-info/diagnosis/blackouts-checklist. A North American version, the Fainting Checklist, is available from www.stars-us.org/patient-information/fainting_checklist. The Checklist Information Booklet is also available on these sites (**Box 5**).

BLACKOUTS CHECKLIST

The Blackouts Checklist was prepared under the guidance of the STARS expert Medical Advisory Committee. Its principal aim is to help you and your doctor reach the correct diagnosis for any unexplained loss of consciousness (blackout).

The Checklist gives you information and advice on the major reasons for experiencing a blackout, helps you prepare for a doctor's appointment, and provides information on what to expect if you have to attend a hospital appointment.

Checklist: What Do You Need to Know?

A blackout is a temporary loss of consciousness

If someone loses consciousness for a few seconds or minutes, they are often said to have had a blackout.

Every patient presenting with an unexplained blackout should be given a 12-lead ECG (heart rhythm check)

It is important that the ECG is passed as normal.

Most unexplained blackouts are caused by syncope

Many people, including doctors, assume that blackouts are due to epileptic seizures, but much more commonly they are due to syncope (pronounced sin-co-pee), a type of blackout that is caused by a problem in the regulation of blood pressure or sometimes in the heart. Up to 40% of the population will lose consciousness at some point in their life due to syncope. Syncope can affect all age groups but the causes vary with age, and in older adults multiple causes often exist.

Many syncopal attacks only require reassurance from your GP

Many syncopal attacks require only explanation and reassurance from a GP or trained nurse regarding the likely absence of anything being seriously wrong. Consultation with a specialist will be necessary, however, if the cause of the syncope remains uncertain or if there are symptoms causing particular concern or there is a family history of a heart condition.

There are three major reasons why people may experience a blackout(s)

- **Syncope: a sudden lack of blood supply to the brain.** Syncope is caused by a problem in the regulation of blood pressure or a problem with the heart.
- **Epilepsy: an electrical short-circuiting in the brain.** Epileptic attacks are usually called seizures. Diagnosis of epilepsy is made by a neurologist.
- **Psychogenic blackouts: resulting from stress or anxiety.** Psychogenic blackouts occur most often in young adults. They may be difficult to diagnose. Psychogenic does not mean that people are putting it on. However, there is often underlying stress caused by extreme pressure at school or work. In exceptional cases, some people may have experienced ill treatment or abuse in childhood.

Misdiagnosis is common but avoidable

- Many syncopal attacks are mistaken for epilepsy.
- However, epilepsy affects less than 1% of the population.
- UK research has shown that approximately 30% of adults and up to 40% of children diagnosed with epilepsy in the United Kingdom do not have the condition.
- Many elements of a syncopal attack, such as random jerking of limbs, are similar to those experienced during an epileptic seizure.
- It can be difficult to differentiate the causes of the blackout.

Syncope causes falls

- Syncope causes a significant number of falls in older adults, particularly when the falls are sudden and not obviously the result of a trip or slip.
- Many older adults only recall a fall and do not realize they have blacked out.

- Greater awareness of syncope as a cause of falls is key to effective treatment and prevention of recurring falls.

Since originally launched in 2006 by Sir Roger Moore (aka James Bond!), who has syncope, demand for the Checklist has been undiminished. It won an award from the British Medical Association and continues to be the most widely distributed (and online accessed) item of patient literature produced by STARS.

This focus on the empowerment of patients has helped fill an important gap in patient care, and has greatly improved the perspective a patient can expect to develop toward syncope.

And our Family?

In 2009, STARS received recognition. I was awarded the Member of the British Empire (MBE) medal by Her Majesty the Queen for services to health care.

My daughter is now 23 years old and works full-time for STARS. She still occasionally experiences reflex syncope and the fear of injuring herself during a blackout. Only this week she fainted and subsequently broke her arm during the fall. Throughout school and university, teachers and fellow students were informed as to what action to take when she fell unconscious to the ground (make her safe, place a hand on her and keep telling her she will be OK. She tells me that this helps as she begins to regain consciousness, knowing she is not alone). I attended more birthday parties, school trips, and swimming classes than any other mother I know. My daughter was not allowed to participate unless I was present because the teachers would not take responsibility for her well-being. It took more than a year before a driving license was granted.

My eldest daughter has also experienced episodes of fainting. She is now a qualified doctor. I often think the work she has done for STARS over the years and listening to patients' stories led her to this career.

And my husband? One morning in 2008 he turned to me and said "Trudie I am going to faint"; with that he fell to the floor dead.

There is no such thing as a simple faint.

REFERENCES

1. Moya A, Sutton R, Ammirati F, et al. Guidelines for the diagnosis and management of syncope (version 2009): the Task Force for the Diagnosis and Management of Syncope of the European Society of Cardiology (ESC). Eur Heart J 2009;30(21):2631–71.
2. Thijs RD, Wieling W, Kaufmann H, et al. Defining and classifying syncope. Clin Auton Res 2004; 14(Suppl 1):4–8.
3. van Dijk JG, Thijs RD, Benditt DG, et al. A guide to disorders causing transient loss of consciousness: focus on syncope. Nat Rev Neurol 2009;5(8):438–48.
4. Soteriades ES, Evans JC, Larson MG, et al. Incidence and prognosis of syncope. N Engl J Med 2002;347(12):878–85.
5. Ganzeboom KS, Colman N, Reitsma JB, et al. Prevalence and triggers of syncope in medical students. Am J Cardiol 2003;91(8):1006–8.
6. Brignole M, Alboni P, Benditt DG, et al. Guidelines on management (diagnosis and treatment) of syncope—update 2004. Europace 2004;6(6):467–537.
7. Rose MS, Koshman ML, Spreng S, et al. The relationship between health-related quality of life and frequency of spells in patients with syncope. J Clin Epidemiol 2000;53:1209–16.
8. Van Dijk N, Boer KR, Colman N, et al. High diagnostic yield and accuracy of history, physical examination, and ECG in patients with transient loss of consciousness in FAST: the Fainting Assessment study. J Cardiovasc Electrophysiol 2008;19(1):48–55.
9. Gulamhusein S, Naccarelli GV, Ko PT, et al. Value and limitations of clinical electrophysiologic study in assessment of patients with unexplained syncope. Am J Med 1982;73:700–5.
10. Zaidi A, Clough P, Cooper P, et al. Misdiagnosis of epilepsy: many seizure-like attacks have a cardiovascular cause. J Am Coll Cardiol 2000;36(1):181–4.
11. Zubcevic S, Gavranovic M, Catibusic F, et al. Frequency of misdiagnosis of epilepsy in a group of 79 children with diagnosis of intractable epilepsy. Proceedings of International League Against Epilepsy [abstract: 337]. 2001.
12. Uldall P, Alving J, Buchholt J, et al. Evaluation of a tertiary referral epilepsy centre for children. Proceedings of International League Against Epilepsy [abstract]. 2001. p. 146.

Approach to the Patient with Syncope
Venues, Presentations, Diagnoses

David G. Benditt, MD*, Wayne O. Adkisson, MD

KEYWORDS

• Syncope • Classification • Presentation • Diagnoses

KEY POINTS

• When a patient presents with syncope, the physician's key tasks are to establish a confident causal diagnosis, assess prognostic implications, and provide appropriate advice to prevent recurrences.
• It is important to develop an organized approach to the assessment of the patient with syncope, including a careful initial examination as well as application of specialized syncope evaluation units and structured questionnaires for history taking.
• The initial patient evaluation, particularly a detailed medical history, is the key to identifying the most likely diagnosis.
• Carefully selected diagnostic tests can be chosen to confirm the clinical suspicion.

INTRODUCTION

Syncope is a syndrome in which a brief and self-limited period of loss of consciousness is triggered by transient insufficiency of oxygen delivery to the brain[1–4]; most often syncope is caused by a self-limited period of systemic hypotension, resulting in reduced cerebral blood flow.

A wide range of conditions may be responsible for initiating syncope (**Fig. 1**):

• In many instances the cause is relatively benign from a mortality perspective, such as,
  ○ Assumption of upright posture in patients susceptible to orthostatic faints
  ○ Emotional upset or pain, causing a vaso-vagal faint
  ○ Coughing in patients susceptible to cough syncope
  ○ Emptying the bladder in postmicturition syncope, and so forth.

• In other cases, the basis for the faint may be caused by a more serious problem, such as
  ○ Sinus arrest/pause
  ○ Atrioventricular (AV) block
  ○ Ventricular tachyarrhythmias.

Whether the basis for symptoms is innocent or potentially life-threatening, syncope may lead to physical injury, accidents that put the affected individual and others at risk, and impaired quality of life (QoL).[1]

In economic terms, the Ambulatory and Hospital Care Statistics Branch of the Centers for Disease Control and Prevention's National Center for Health Statistics periodically provides (http://www.cdc.gov/nchs/ahcd.htm) nationally representative data on ambulatory care visits to hospital emergency departments (EDs) in the United States. Statistics are based on data collected in the National Hospital Ambulatory Medical Care Survey (NHAMCS). NHAMCS is a national probability survey of ED

Cardiovascular Division, Department of Medicine, Cardiac Arrhythmia and Syncope Center, University of Minnesota Medical School, 420 Delaware Street South East, Minneapolis, MN 55455, USA
* Corresponding author. Mail Code 508, 420 Delaware Street Southeast, Minneapolis, MN 55455.
E-mail address: bendi001@umn.edu

Cardiol Clin 31 (2013) 9–25
http://dx.doi.org/10.1016/j.ccl.2012.09.002

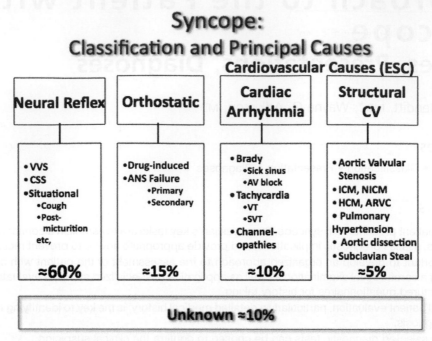

Fig. 1. A commonly used classification of the causes of syncope.

visits and outpatient departments of nonfederal short-stay and general hospitals in the United States. The NHAMCS in 2006 noted that primary diagnosis of syncope and collapse (*International Classification of Diseases, Ninth Revision*; 780.2) had increased from approximately 887,000 ED visits in 2001 to greater than 1,125,000 ED visits in 2006. In 2008, syncope and collapse remained in the top 10 reasons for ED visits for both men and women.

The direct costs and indirect (eg, lost productivity) economic implications of syncope and collapse are substantial (**Box 1**).[5,6] In terms of direct costs, the in-hospital expenses comprise the major portion, and these costs are largely driven by physician's tendency to admit patients with syncope for evaluation. It is thought that many of these admissions could be avoided and the evaluations undertaken in a less costly outpatient environment. Standardizing history taking and development of precise risk stratification methods for patients with syncope may help in this regard[1,7,8]; however, optimal tools for this purpose have yet to be developed.[9,10]

In addition to financial issues, recurrent syncope has serious effects on QoL. Lifestyle impairment because of syncope is comparable with that associated with chronic illnesses such as arthritis, depressive disorders, and renal disease. Psychosocial impairment has an estimated average adverse impact on QoL of 33% on daily life, similar to that caused by epilepsy.[1,11,12]

Given the multiple adverse implications of syncope and collapse in terms of individual health and economic impact, prevention is important. Prevention can be achieved only if the specific cause of the faint is identified, and thereafter, an effective treatment plan designed to prevent recurrences is instituted.[1]

VENUES

The frequency with which syncope occurs has been assessed in a variety of studies. In general, the reported prevalence of syncope, which to be more precise reflects the percentage of individuals who have experienced a faint, varies widely; in large part, differences are attributable to the nature of the population being evaluated.

EDs (and in recent years urgent-care clinics) are often the first places that fainters come to for attention. In these settings, syncope and collapse are estimated to account for approximately 1% of visits in Europe, and from 1% to 6% in the United States.[1,10,13–17]

Studies based on recollection of syncope events provide a wide range when trying to estimate the percentage of individuals who have experienced at least 1 episode of syncope.[18–25] By way of example, an early report from the Framingham follow-up study[18] found that only 3.2% of adults admitted to 1 or more syncope spells. The first syncope occurred at an average age of 52 years

---

Box 1
Direct cost estimated economic implications of syncope and collapse

1. US data derived from the US Medicare database, 2000.[5]

   a. Direct cost estimates

   b. Estimated total annual charges for syncope-related admissions: $5.4 billion (95% confidence interval [CI] $4.9–$6.0 billion)

   c. Mean charge: $12,000 (95% CI $11,000–$12,000) per hospitalization

   d. Estimated total annual costs for syncope-related admissions were $2.4 billion (95% CI $2.2–$2.6 billion)

   e. Mean cost of $5400 (95% CI $5100–$5600) per hospitalization

2. UK data for 2005 to 2006

   a. Average cost of £836 (US$1600) per patient

   b. £70 million (US $135 million) per annum

   c. About 17% of falls in elderly people are caused by syncope complicated by fractures; the cost exceeds £1 billion

3. Spain (tertiary-care hospital)[6]

   a. Diagnosis of vasovagal syncope during hospitalization was the least expensive (approximately $2000)

   b. Syncope secondary to cardiac ischemia was more expensive (approximately $7000)

   c. Syncope secondary to ventricular arrhythmias was the most expensive; diagnostic test amounted to €3577 (about $4650) and therapeutic procedures cost €23,115 (approximately $30,000)

   d. Costs escalated further when syncope was recurrent and unexplained

      i. Mean annual cost at the first hospitalization was about $3390 (standard deviation [SD] $3246)

      ii. A further increase of cost was noted if a second hospitalization $5281 (SD $4424) was needed

---

(range 17–78 years) for men, and 50 years (range 13–87 years) for women. In addition, although syncope occurred at virtually all ages, syncope burden tended to increase with advancing age from 8/1000 person-examinations in the 35-year-old to 44-year-old age group to approximately 40/1000 person-examinations in the 75-year-old and older age group. However, a subsequent assessment of the Framingham data[19] indicated that 10% of 7814 patients admitted to at least 1 syncope spell over a 17-year sampling time, a higher number than in the original report.

In another extensive community-based study of US adults aged 45 years or older, Chen and colleagues[20] reported that 19% of adults admitted to at least 1 syncope spell. More recently, studies from Calgary, Canada and Amsterdam, The Netherlands reported similar results for estimates of community lifetime cumulative incidence. Ganzeboom and colleagues[22] surveyed medical students and found that 39% had fainted at least once. The Calgary group[21,23] reported that the likelihood of at least 1 faint was 37% by age 60 years, and almost all first spells occurred by age 40 years. Further, the Calgary findings indicated that by age 60 years, 31% of men and 42% of

women had fainted, similar to the proportions reported by the Amsterdam study.[22]

In terms of populations enrolled in more structured care studies, Ungar and colleagues reported 2-year follow-up in the Evaluation of Guidelines in Syncope Study 2 (EGSYS2) study.[25] Of the original 465 patients included in this 11-hospital Italian study, complete follow-up was available in 86%. Despite treatment, syncope recurrence occurred in 16.5% of follow-up patients by 2 years. Death occurred in 9.2% of follow-up patients by 2 years, of which one-fourth were considered cardiovascular. Mortality risk was associated (univariate) with:

- Age
- Fewer syncope events
- Abnormal electrocardiogram (ECG)
- Presence of heart disease
- Trauma

In more discrete population sets, syncope has been estimated to occur in[1,24,25]:

- 15% of children younger than 18 years
- 25% of young military population
- Up to 23% of a nursing home population older than 70 years

With respect to elderly patients, the reported frequency of syncope may be an underestimate because many of these individuals show various degrees of cognitive impairment that affect memory of events; up to 20% of these individuals are believed to be amnestic for such episodes (ie, retrograde amnesia) and often when queried deny that they ever lost consciousness.

Taken together, the various memory-based studies suggest that roughly 20% to 40% of people report having fainted at least once in their lives. Women and younger individuals may be more susceptible, or more honest, or simply have better memories. Further, the syncope recurrence rate seems to be high. Within 3 years of the initial episode, on average about 35% of patients experience recurrences.

PRESENTATIONS
Pathophysiology

As noted earlier, transient global cerebral hypoperfusion is the essential feature of syncope pathophysiology.[1–3] In most cases, diminished cerebral perfusion is caused by a transient decrease in systemic blood pressure.

Acute hypoxemia, such as might occur with abrupt high-altitude aircraft decompression, could also be the culpable trigger, but is rare. However, more common medical conditions that inherently reduce oxygen delivery to the brain (eg, anemia, obstructive airway disease, high altitude) increase susceptibility to syncope, Thus, in these circumstances, lesser degrees of hypotension may initiate a faint that otherwise might not have occurred.

Loss of postural tone is an inevitable consequence of loss of consciousness. If the affected individual is not restrained, they slump to a gravitationally neutral position (eg, fall to the ground). On occasion, the victim may have jerky movements after onset of loss of consciousness; because of these muscle movements, true syncope may be mistaken for a seizure disorder or fit by untrained witnesses.[3] Sometimes, nonskeletal smooth muscle function may be affected, resulting in loss of bladder (common) or bowel (rare) control and further raising concern that the patient had experienced an epileptic seizure.[3]

Cause

In terms of the causes of syncope, younger patients without structural heart disease tend to be mainly affected by neurally mediated reflex faints, and especially vasovagal syncope.[1,4,20–23] However, although rare compared with reflex faints in this seemingly otherwise healthy population, the possibility of a so-called channelopathy (eg, long QT syndrome, Brugada syndrome, catecholaminergic paroxysmal ventricular tachycardia [VT]) should not be overlooked, particularly if the history is not typical for reflex syncope. Channelopathies are being recognized with increasing frequency and may have a worrisome prognosis; some remain as yet unidentified from a genetic perspective but nevertheless can cause life-threatening arrhythmias.[1,26,27]

There should also be increased concern for more worrisome causes of syncope (eg, cardiac arrhythmias, orthostatic faints caused by primary neurologic disease) among patients with known or suspected structural cardiovascular disease, such as:

- Coronary artery disease
- Valvular heart disease
- Cardiomyopathies
- Hypertensive heart disease
- Congenital heart disease, including previously operated congenital conditions
- Elderly individuals

Mortality is a greater concern in patients with than in those without structural disease; however, in most cases, the primary mortality driver is the severity of the heart disease rather than the syncope itself.[1] Further, whatever the cause of syncope, older patients with faints are at increased risk of serious injury.[1,3,21,22,25]

In a study of 242 older individuals aged 65 to 98 years, Ungar and colleagues[28] found that the combination of neural reflex and orthostatic faints accounted for 67% of diagnoses. Vasovagal, situational, and carotid sinus syndrome (CSS) (ie, the neurally mediated reflex faints) made up 62% of cases in patients 75 years and younger and 36% in patients older than 75 years. More recently, Anapalahan and Gibson[29] reported observations in 200 patients 65 years or older who presented to the ED because of unexplained or accidental falls. These investigators' findings indicated that approximately 25% of unexplained falls were caused by neurally mediated reflex syncope.

Orthostatic faints and CSS are particularly prevalent in older patients.[1,13,14,28,30] In the case of orthostatic faints, age-related neurologic causes including subtle forms of Parkinson disease or autonomic failure contribute importantly to syncope susceptibility. However, drug-induced orthostatic hypotension should not be overlooked, because it is common and often readily managed.

CSS has been reported to account for ~20% of syncope in older individuals, with vasovagal syncope amounting to a further 15%. Although less frequent, cardiac causes become more important with increasing age and the inevitable greater concomitant prevalence of structural heart disease.[1]

DIAGNOSIS: STRATEGY AND SPECIFIC CLINICAL CONSIDERATIONS
Strategy

Fig. 2 provides an overview of a recommended approach to the assessment of a patient who presents with an apparent episode of transient loss of consciousness (T-LOC)/collapse based on the European Society of Cardiology Syncope Task Force Guidelines.[1] Box 2 summarizes clinical features of a faint that may help to suggest a cause. However, although these features may be helpful in a general sense, they should not be relied on on their own; a careful assessment of each patient by an experienced clinician, preferably using a thorough structured interview instrument is essential.

The urgency of determining the basis of syncope is determined by assessment of the patient's short-term and long-term potential morbidity and mortality risk. This risk-assessment step has received considerable attention recently.[1,9,17,31–38] Its importance relates only in part to potential for death in such patients but also to susceptibility for syncope to recur in

affected individuals and result in falls with injury, and economic and lifestyle disruption. As noted earlier, it is estimated that about one-third of patients with syncope have recurrences by 3 years of follow-up,[1] with the bulk of these recurrences occurring within the first 2 years.

Strong predictors of a greater risk of syncope (or apparent syncope) recurrence include a history of recurrent syncope at the time of presentation (ie, recurrences, at least statistically, tend to lead to more future recurrences), age younger than 45 years, or a psychiatric diagnosis. After positive tilt-table testing, patients with a past history of more than 6 syncope spells have a risk of recurrence of more than 50% over 2 years.[1,29] In addition, in a more recent analysis that mainly included a young referral-based population, a history of syncope in the past year (ie, before the presenting event) was shown to better predict recurrent syncope than was a history of syncope in the more distant past.[39]

A few studies have attempted to identify clinical factors associated with high risk of mortality or symptom recurrence in patients presenting to the ED with syncope and collapse.[9,10,13,17,31–38] For the most part, the studies have focused on the short-term horizon (ie, 7 days to 1 month) to ascertain which patients are best hospitalized immediately for evaluation, and which can be sent

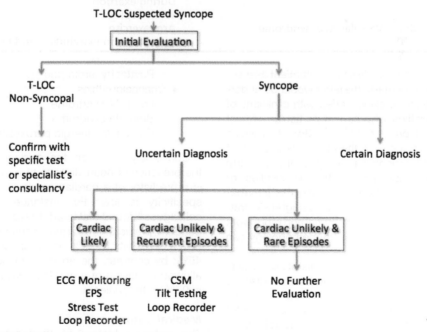

Fig. 2. The general strategy for evaluation of syncope as recommended in the European Society of Cardiology Syncope Practice Guidelines. See text for discussion. T-LOC, transient loss of consciousness. (Data from Moya A, Sutton R, Ammirati F, et al. Task Force for the Diagnosis and Management of Syncope, European Society of Cardiology (ESC), European Heart Rhythm Association (EHRA), Heart Failure Association (HFA), Heart Rhythm Society (HRS). For the diagnosis and management of syncope (version 2009). Eur Heart J 2009;30(21):2631–71.)

Box 2
Clinical features that may suggest a cause of syncope

Cause	Subtype	Clinical Features
Neural reflex syncope	Vasovagal faint	No structural cardiovascular disease Long history of recurrent faints After unexpected emotional distress, pain Hot crowded environment Warning symptoms of feeling hot/cold Nausea After a meal Postevent fatigue
	CSS	Older (usually male) Turning/stretching neck
	Cardioinhibitory	
	Vasodepressor	
	Mixed	
	Situational faint	After specific actions
	Postmicturition	
	Cough	
	Defecation	
	Swallow, and so forth	
Orthostatic syncope	Immediate (occurs immediately after standing up, may occur in healthy individuals)	After moving from lying or seated to standing (may be delayed) Presence of neurodisease
	Delayed or classic (occurs sometimes several minutes after standing up)	(eg, Parkinsonism, diabetes) Drugs that promote vasodilation or diuresis
Cardiac syncope		Structural heart disease or channelopathy present During exertion While supine
Cerebrovascular	Vascular steal syndrome	Arm exercise Differences in extremity blood pressure

home with a plan for early timely outpatient assessment (**Box 3**). Optimally, the latter would be undertaken in a syncope clinic staffed with clinicians of various specialties who have a particular interest in this clinical problem.[1,7,8,10,17] **Box 3** provides a summary of some of the clinical features that have proved worrisome in analysis of short-term risk after syncope presentation in studies or consensus documents. In reviewing this information, it should be understood that no single risk stratification scheme has proved optimal and more work remains before a consensus on methodology can be derived.

The absence of a past medical history of cardiac disease and signs of structural heart disease (including ECG and often echocardiographic assessment) largely excludes a cardiac cause for syncope.[1,34,40] However, there are several important exceptions:

- Paroxysmal supraventricular tachycardia (SVT), including:
  - Preexcitation syndromes
  - Posttachycardia pauses
- Channelopathies
  - Long QT syndrome
  - Brugada syndrome
  - Catecholaminergic paroxysmal VT

Conversely, although the evidence indicating the presence of heart disease at initial evaluation is a predictor of a cardiac cause of syncope, its specificity is low. For instance, Alboni and colleagues[40] found that heart disease was an independent predictor of cardiac cause of syncope, with a sensitivity of 95% and a specificity of only 45%; by contrast, the absence of heart disease allowed exclusion of a cardiac cause of syncope in 97% of the patients.

Medical history

The patient's history of their symptoms and witnesses' accounts often reveals the most likely cause of the collapse and thereby guides subsequent evaluation. However, the history taking must be thorough to be of value, and should

Box 3
Clinical features used in selected short-term syncope risk stratification studies

Study	Risk Horizon	Clinical High-Risk Markers
San Francisco Rule[32]	1 week	Abnormal ECG (nonsinus rhythm or new abnormality)
		CHF
		Shortness of breath
		Hypotension (systolic <90 mm Hg)
		Hematocrit less than 30%
ROSE rule[35]	1 month	Abnormal ECG
		Increased brain natriuretic peptide
		Chest pain
		Fecal blood
SEEDS[31]		Abnormal ECG/cardiac monitor (signs of ischemia, atrial fibrillation, VT, permanent pacemaker/implantable cardioverter defibrillator dysfunction, long QT, marked bradycardia)
		Chest pain compatible with acute coronary syndrome
		CHF
		Valvular heart disease
STePs[36]	10 days	Abnormal ECG
		Trauma
		No warning
		Male gender
OESIL[38]	12 months	Abnormal ECG
		Age older than 65 years
		History of cardiovascular disease
		No warning

Abbreviation: CHF, congestive heart failure.

carefully encompass not only the index presentation but also previous events, associated symptoms, comorbid conditions, drug/dietary issues, and family/genetic aspects.[1,34] In this regard, a pre-prepared history form may facilitate the recording of the complete picture. Structured questionnaires can be helpful in preventing valuable information from being overlooked. However, as pointed out by Colman and colleagues,[34] the structured approach may be most useful in the ED or the urgent-care clinic, and of lesser value in specialized syncope clinics, where the more difficult cases require experienced practitioners looking for more subtle findings.

The essential key questions to be determined early in the evaluation process are:

- Is loss of consciousness attributable to true syncope versus other causes, including accidental falls?
- Is heart disease present?
- Are there important clinical features in the history that suggest the diagnosis (eg, premonitory symptoms in vasovagal fainters)?

A comprehensive discussion of history taking in the patient with syncope lies beyond the scope of

this article. Nonetheless, several reports provide insight into the usefulness of careful history taking (usually in conjunction with physical examination) in establishing a working diagnosis for the basis of syncope. Overall, a diagnosis is reported to have been obtained in this manner in roughly 30% to 70% of patients.[1,34,41–46] Some studies primarily addressed specific issues (eg, diagnosing vasovagal syncope), whereas others have examined broader problems, such as differentiating syncope from seizures, or identifying clinical markers suggesting cardiac syncope. For example:

- Alboni and colleagues[40] used a standard comprehensive questionnaire in the evaluation of 341 (average age 61 ± 20 years; approximately equal men and women) consecutive patients with syncope referred to specialized syncope units. The medical history alone was deemed to provide a diagnosis in 14% of cases. However, when other aspects of the initial evaluation were included (eg, ECG, carotid massage, orthostatic blood pressure measurement), the diagnostic yield increased to 40%.
- Sarasin and colleagues[41] used a standardized approach (ie, history questionnaire, physical examination, ECG, and orthostatic

blood pressures) for the syncope diagnosis in 650 consecutive patients (age 60 ± 23 years; approximately equal men and women) seen in the ED. In almost 70% of cases, the investigators reported that a sufficiently strong basis for a syncope diagnosis was established (reflex syncope, 36%; orthostatic syncope, 24%, cardiac arrhythmia or acute ischemia, 5%; other, 3%).

- Oh and colleagues[42] primarily addressed the distinction between reflex and cardiac syncope in 497 patients (mean age 53 years) referred to an academic center. However, in terms of the value of history and physical examination for establishing a diagnosis, the investigators identified reflex or orthostatic syncope in 40% of cases, and other causes in 5%. Thus a strong diagnostic suspicion was established in 45% of cases.
- Sheldon and colleagues[43] addressed the issue of differentiating syncope from seizures by a historical features scoring system. This method was successful in terms of distinguishing these 2 key clinical problems. The same investigators later offered a similar scoring approach (Calgary Syncope Score) to differentiate vasovagal syncope from other causes of T-LOC (**Table 1**). The validity of the Calgary Syncope Score has been the subject of independent assessment; Romme and colleagues[44] from Amsterdam evaluated the Calgary Syncope Score in a cohort of 503 patients with syncope. The sensitivity for making a vasovagal diagnosis by this method was confirmed (87%; 95% CI: 82%–91%) in the

overall group and 92% (95% CI: 86%–95%) in younger patients less than 50 years of age. However, overall specificity was disappointingly low at 32%. In addition, preliminary findings from the Calgary group suggest that the score may be less precise in older patients (>60 years) compared with younger individuals.

Physical findings

Most patients with presumed syncope have fully recovered by the time they are first seen by a medical practitioner in the emergency room or urgent-care clinic. Consequently, the relation between physical finding abnormalities (if any) and the cause of syncope is at best inferential.

Physical findings that may help to establish a basis for syncope include orthostatic blood pressure changes, cardiac murmurs or bruits, and an abnormal response to carotid sinus message; the last being a recommended diagnostic step during the physical examination, especially in the older person (>60 years). Additional findings from the ECG, echocardiogram, chest radiograph, and blood count may also be reasonably incorporated in the initial evaluation process.

Signs of new focal neurologic lesions, such as hemiparesis, dysarthria, diplopia, and vertigo may reasonably suggest that a reported collapse was not true syncope, but rather a primary neurologic problem; however, this is not a concrete rule. For instance, signs of Parkinsonism or severe autonomic disease may be suggestive of a possible orthostatic faint (and the history should be revisited carefully to ascertain if it is supportive of such a diagnosis).

Table 1	
Calgary scoring system for vasovagal syncope	
Question	**Points (If Yes)**
1. History of any one of bifascicular block, asystole, SVT, diabetes	−5 points
2. Have bystanders noted you to be blue during the faint?	−4 points
3. Did syncope start at age >35 y?	−3 points
4. Do you remember anything about being unconscious?	−2 points
5. Do you have lightheaded spells or faints with prolonged standing or sitting?	+1 point
6. Do you feel warm before your faint?	+2 points
7. Do you have lightheaded spells or faints with pain or in a medical setting?	+3 points
	Sum of above = total point score
Vasovagal syncope if total score ≥2	
Excluded patients: known cardiomyopathy or myocardial infarction	

Data from Sheldon R, Rose S, Connolly S, et al. Diagnostic criteria for vasovagal syncope based on a quantitative history. Eur Heart J 2006;27(3):344–50.

Diagnostic yield

Pooled data from population-based studies indicate that the history and physical examination identify a potential cause of syncope in approximately 40% of the patients.[1,17,20,28,34,40,45,46] Reflex syncope (vasovagal, situational) account for approximately 75% of diagnoses at initial evaluation. The diagnostic yield of standard ECG obtained in the ED is, on average 6% and accounts for about half of total diagnoses of cardiac syncope. In-hospital (telemetry) monitoring is helpful in a few selected high-risk patients.[47]

Routine blood tests rarely yield diagnostically useful information. In selected syncope cases, they can confirm a clinical suspicion of acute anemia, acute myocardial infarction, or pulmonary embolism. Rarely, such tests may yield other non-syncope diagnoses such as hypoglycemia and intoxications.

Neurologic studies, such as electroencephalogram (EEG), carotid Doppler recordings, or head magnetic resonance imaging (MRI)/computed tomography (CT) are almost never of value.[1,4] They should be restricted to those cases in which head injury may have occurred as a result of a collapse, or the patient is believed to have had a seizure (ie, not syncope), or there are new localizing neurologic signs present on examination.

SPECIFIC DIAGNOSES
Neurally Mediated Reflex Syncope

Neurally mediated reflex faints (often simply termed reflex faints) are the most common cause of syncope when all age groups and presentations are considered.[1] The most frequently occurring forms of the reflex faints are vasovagal syncope and CSS. Situational syncope (eg, postmicturition syncope, defecation syncope, swallow syncope, cough syncope) is also encountered from time to time, but in these cases the history is generally sufficient to establish the diagnosis, and from a practical perspective they may be considered special cases of the vasovagal faint.[48]

Tilt-table testing, carotid sinus massage (CSM), and other assessments of autonomic function (eg, baroreceptor sensitivity, heart rate variability) are occasionally used for assessment of patients with suspected reflex syncope.[1,48–57] However, except for tilt testing in the case of vasovagal faints, and carotid massage in suspected CSS,[1,49] the clinical value of other tests is unclear and they play little role in clinical decision making.

In terms of other tests, as noted earlier, neurologic studies (head MRI or CT scans, as well as EEGs) are often ordered by physicians for syncope evaluation, but usually are a waste of resources and contribute little to the diagnosis, especially in the case of neural reflex syncope.[1] The adenosine triphosphate test remains a controversial topic.[55–57] It may have a role to play in the older fainter, in whom neural reflex mechanisms may be relevant but are difficult to unmask.

Vasovagal syncope

Vasovagal syncope usually occurs sporadically, and may affect 10% to 20% of the general population during their lifetime. This form of syncope (also termed the common faint) is often encountered in young otherwise healthy patients, but may occur in all age groups, and is generally unassociated with cardiovascular or neurologic diseases. However, there is no rule that precludes patients with structural cardiovascular disease from experiencing a vasovagal faint, and the clinical picture can be variable.[1]

Vasovagal syncope may be triggered in a variety of ways, including unpleasant sights, pain, extreme emotion, and prolonged standing. However, not infrequently, the precise trigger for a given symptomatic event remains unknown. Autonomic activation (eg, flushing and sweating) in the premonitory phase strongly suggests a vasovagal origin. Typical presentations occur in about 40% of presumed vasovagal syncope, but less often in older patients. In cases in which the presentation is not classic but in which vasovagal syncope is a possible cause, a head-up tilt-table test is often used to help support the diagnosis.

Head-up tilt testing, although imperfect in terms of diagnostic precision, is the only laboratory test deemed useful in diagnosing vasovagal syncope. Insertable loop recorders (ILRs) may also be helpful, and are of particular value for documenting spontaneous events, particularly if there is a prominent cardioinhibitory component to the event. However, in cases of a predominantly vasodepressor form of reflex syncope, the variation of heart rate detected by the ILR may be subtle; it may be difficult to discern whether a vasovagal event occurred.

The head-up tilt-table test in a drug-free state seems to discriminate well between symptomatic patients and asymptomatic control individuals.[1,51] The false-positive rate of the tilt test is approximately 10%. Test sensitivity seems to be increased with the use of pharmacologic provocation (isoproterenol or nitroglycerin), but at the cost of reduced specificity.[52–54] For patients without severe structural heart disease, a positive tilt-table test (especially if it reproduces the patient's spontaneous symptoms) can be considered diagnostic. On the other hand, for patients with significant structural heart disease, other more serious causes of syncope must be excluded before relying on a positive tilt test result.

Complete review of treatment approaches to vasovagal syncope has been provided elsewhere.[1,58] However, in most cases of vasovagal syncope, patients principally require reassurance and education regarding the nature of the condition. In patients with multiple recurrent syncope, initial advice should include review of the types of environments in which syncope is more common (eg, hot, crowded, and emotionally upsetting situations) and provide insight into the typical warning symptoms (eg, hot/cold feeling, sweaty, clammy, nauseated), which may permit many individuals to recognize and respond to an impending episode and thereby avert the faint. Additional common sense measures, such as keeping well hydrated (especially with electrolyte-rich beverages), and avoiding prolonged exposure to upright posture or hot confining environments, should also be discussed.

Many drugs have been proposed for treatment of vasovagal syncope (eg, β-blockers, disopyramide, midodrine, serotonin inhibitors). However, placebo-controlled trials have generally not shown a benefit.[1] The principal exception may be midodrine, a vasoconstrictor agent (although even with this agent data are conflicting),[59–61] and perhaps fludrocortisone.

The role of cardiac pacing for vasovagal syncope remains controversial as well. Recently, however, both the ISSUE 2 and ISSUE 3 trials have suggested that cardiac pacing may be useful in selected older patients in whom a prolonged asystole has been documented during spontaneous (as opposed to tilt-table–triggered) vasovagal events.[62,63] As a rule, ILR confirmation of clinically significant bradycardia or asystole is necessary to make the case for pacing. Further, the existing data supporting pacing apply only to an older population averaging around 60 years of age; marked asystole in young patients should not be considered an immediate pacemaker indication given the long-term implications of such a decision.

CSS

CSS tends to occur most often in older men, and is especially associated with concomitant atherosclerotic disease. Spontaneous CSS accounts for about 1% of all causes of syncope, and may be defined as syncope that seems to occur in close relationship with accidental mechanical manipulation of the neck.[49,63–69] It is presumed that the basis for the faint is mediated through the carotid sinus baroreceptors, but disturbances of neck proprioception may contribute.[65]

Diagnostic testing provides the strongest evidence in favor of CSS when symptoms are reproduced by CSM,[1,68] usually in conjunction with a period of asystole, paroxysmal AV block, or a marked decrease (usually >50 mm Hg systolic) in systemic arterial pressure. In many instances, the most convincing results from CSM are obtained when massage is undertaken in the upright position. An alternative, albeit less specific approach is defined as a CSM-induced ventricular pause of 3 seconds or longer or a decrease of systolic blood pressure 50 mm Hg or greater.[1]

Treatment of CSS is guided by assessment of the relative importance of cardioinhibitory versus vasodepressor physiology[69]; for the most part, this assessment is best made by undertaking CSM under various patient conditions:

- Resting flat
- During upright posture, usually on a tilt table at 70°
- During temporary cardiac pacing to evaluate the hypotensive response independent of induced bradycardia

In general, cardiac pacing seems to be beneficial and is acknowledged to be the treatment of choice when marked bradycardia has been documented. Judicious use of vasoconstrictors (eg, midodrine) may be needed for patients in whom the vasodepressor aspect of the reflex is prominent.

Situational faints

Situational faints encompass a wide range of clinical scenarios, and are recognized by a careful medical history. Each is characterized by the specific clinical circumstances surrounding (and presumably triggering) the event (eg, cough syncope, micturition syncope, and swallow syncope). Treatment relies heavily on avoidance of triggering circumstances, or at least reducing the risk associated with the circumstance.

Orthostatic Hypotension

Orthostatic syncope can be diagnosed when there is documentation of posturally induced hypotension associated with syncope or presyncope.[1,70–72] Two forms are recognized: (1) the immediate form occurs almost immediately after the patient stands up, and then disappears quickly, (2) the classic or delayed form is defined as a decline in systolic blood pressure of at least 20 mm Hg within 3 to 5 minutes of assuming a standing posture.

It is important to identify nonneurogenic reversible causes of orthostatic hypotension, such as volume depletion, effect of medications (common), and effect of comorbidities (eg, diabetes and alcohol, and more rarely, adrenal insufficiency). Elimination of the responsible drug or offending agent is usually sufficient to improve symptoms.

In some cases, the cause of orthostatic hypotension proves to be a primary neurologic disorder. Parkinsonism is probably the most frequently diagnosed.[1,58,70] Pure autonomic failure is also observed from time to time. Although cure may not be possible, a precise diagnosis can lead to initiation of treatment that may provide substantial symptom relief.

When physical maneuvers and salt/volume repletion alone are not sufficient to suppress symptoms,[1,58,73] pharmacologic interventions may be justified. Fludrocortisone and midodrine are probably the most commonly used drugs for orthostatic hypotension. Fludrocortisone, a synthetic mineralocorticoid with minimal glucocorticoid effect, results in expansion of intravascular and extravascular body fluid. Midodrine is a prodrug that is converted to its active metabolite, desglymidodrine, after absorption.[58–61] It acts on α-adrenoreceptors to cause constriction of both arterial resistance and venous capacitance vessels. For patients with hypertension, supine hypertension is a potential problem during treatment of orthostatic hypotension. In this circumstance, the short half-life of midodrine may offer an advantage over longer-acting fludrocortisone. Patients with supine hypertension are advised to remain upright (sitting or standing) for 4 hours after taking midodrine. In patients with severe supine hypertension,

short-acting antihypertensives, such as captopril, can be given at bedtime. Despite these interventions, it may be necessary in some patients to accept higher resting blood pressures than would normally be considered desirable.

Cardiac Arrhythmias as Primary Cause of Syncope

Both bradycardias and tachycardias can cause syncope; these patients are most appropriately evaluated by a cardiac electrophysiologist.

Bradyarrhythmias

Bradyarrhythmias caused by sinus node dysfunction include sinoatrial bradycardia, sinus pauses, or occasionally asystolic pauses after termination of an atrial tachycardia. Substantiating a spontaneous event is the optimal diagnostic evidence and although difficult, is best achieved using an ECG event recorder or an ILR. In the absence of such correlation, severe sinus bradycardia lower than 40 beats/min or sinus pauses longer than 3 seconds during waking hours are highly suggestive of symptomatic sinus node disease (**Fig. 3**). Pacemaker therapy is usually appropriate.

Chronic or paroxysmal AV block may also be the cause of syncopal episodes.[1] The presence on ECG monitoring of Mobitz II type second-degree AV block, third-degree AV block, or alternating left and right bundle branch block can reasonably be considered diagnostic of a bradycardic cause of syncope.[1] When the diagnosis is uncertain, ambulatory event monitoring (possibility with an

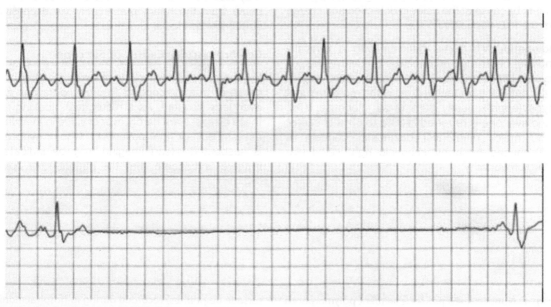

Fig. 3. Abrupt sinus pause of approximately 5 seconds in duration in a 67-year-old man being monitored because of several apparent syncope episodes associated with minor physical trauma.

ILR)[62,63] or electrophysiologic assessment of sinus node and AV conduction with and without pharmacologic challenge may be warranted.[74,75]

Tachyarrhythmias

Although infrequently, SVTs, including atrial flutter or atrial fibrillation, may be associated with syncope at onset of an episode before vascular compensation occurs, or as the result of prolonged bradycardia at the termination of a tachycardia episode. Radiofrequency catheter ablation is the treatment of choice for reentry SVTs or atrial flutter in most patients. A pacemaker may be needed for syncope associated with asystolic pause at termination of supraventricular tachyarrhythmias.

VTs most often occur in patients with structural heart disease, especially ischemic heart disease and dilated cardiomyopathies.[45–48] However, approximately 10% to 15% of patients with VT have no overt structural heart disease.[1,4,25,76–78]

VT associated with ischemic heart disease or dilated cardiomyopathies Ventricular tachyarrhythmias are an important cause of syncope in patients with known structural heart disease.[1,25,76–86] Tachycardia rate, status of left ventricular function, and the efficiency of peripheral vascular constriction determine whether the arrhythmia induces syncopal symptoms. ICDs are the mainstay of treatment of VT associated with structural heart diseases. Pharmacologic therapy and transcatheter ablation are considered principally as adjunctive measures. However, ICD might not prevent faints because of the delay in detection and charge of the ICD capacitor.[80]

Idiopathic VTs Some patients with a clinically normal heart may nonetheless present with idiopathic left ventricular VTs. Idiopathic right ventricular outflow tract tachycardia is the most frequent type (approximately 80% of all idiopathic VTs), and syncope is reported in 23% to 58% of cases. The major differential diagnostic concern is VT caused by arrhythmogenic right ventricular cardiomyopathy.

Less common tachyarrhythmias Other, less common, arrhythmic causes of syncope include left ventricular outflow tract VTs or tachycardias of presumed fascicular origin, ventricular tachyarrhythmias caused by arrhythmogenic right ventricular cardiomyopathy, and torsades de pointes associated with long QT syndromes or Brugada syndrome (**Fig. 4**).[25–27,76–78,86] These conditions are crucial to recognize and are best referred to specialized centers for management, because they are often associated with increased risk of sudden cardiac death.

Structural Cardiac and Cardiopulmonary Causes of Syncope

In these cases, syncope occurs as either a direct result of the structural disturbance or as a consequence of a neural reflex disturbance triggered by the heart condition. Thus, syncope in acute myocardial infarction or severe aortic stenosis may be caused by reduced cardiac output in some cases. Alternatively, neural reflex vasodilation may be triggered and cause hypotension. Probably both mechanisms participate.

In patients with cardiac disease such as hypertrophic cardiomyopathy or aortic stenosis, and apart from any structural-related hemodynamic issues, either SVT or VT may cause cardiac syncope.[87–90] The rapid rates can preclude adequate venous filling in a stiff ventricle, whereas abnormal excitation (especially in VT) may aggravate any tendency for outflow tract obstruction. However, neurally mediated reflex hypotension may also contribute; the triggers are believed to come from the heart, presumably via excessive stretch on ventricular and atrial mechanoreceptors.

Cerebrovascular Causes of Syncope

In general, cerebrovascular diseases are rarely the cause of true syncope.[1,3] Neurologic causes are even less frequent. As a result, tests looking for these diseases are hardly ever of value in the initial assessment of the patient in whom syncope is suspected. Head imaging may be indicated if there is concern that the patient may have

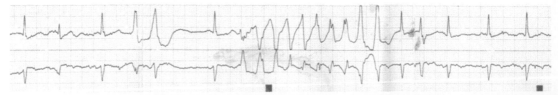

Fig. 4. Nonsustained pause-dependent polymorphous VT (torsade de pointes) recorded during in-hospital monitoring of a patient who presented with syncope, and who had been recently diagnosed with a nonischemic cardiomyopathy and suspected long QT syndrome.

sustained an intracranial injury as a consequence of their collapse.

As a rule, transient ischemic attacks (TIAs) and epilepsy are not part of the differential diagnosis of true syncope. TIAs do not typically cause loss of consciousness, with a rare exception being vertebral-basilar TIAs. Epilepsy is not a form of syncope, but is more reasonably considered in the differential diagnosis of the broader category of conditions that cause T-LOC, of which true syncope is also included.

Cerebrovascular conditions that may be associated with increased susceptibility to true syncope include (in approximate order of frequency, albeit all rare):

1. Migraine (probably via a neural reflex mechanism, particularly vasovagal syncope)
2. Parkinson disease (usually orthostatic)
3. Primary autonomic failure (usually orthostatic or during physical exertion)
4. Subclavian steal syndrome (very rare)

Conditions That Mimic Syncope

Certain medical conditions (**Box 4**) may cause a real or apparent loss of consciousness that might seem to be syncope, but is not true syncope.[3,91] These conditions are important to identify in order for the proper treatment strategy to be initiated; however, they can be time-consuming to pin down.

Whether a particular presentation mimics syncope depends largely on the quality of the account of the events obtained by the physician and their experience in differentiating among these presentations. Most often, an experienced practitioner, after taking a detailed history and interviewing eye-witnesses when possible, can determine whether the episode was a true syncope or not. However, such a distinction is not always possible or accurate. Selected diagnostic testing may yet be required.

Box 4
Common syncope mimics

With impairment or loss of consciousness

  Metabolic disorders, (eg, hypoglycemia, hypoxia, and hyperventilation with hypocapnia)

  Epilepsy

  Intoxication (drugs and alcohol)

  Vertebrobasilar TIA

Without loss of consciousness

  Psychogenic pseudosyncope

  Cataplexy

  Drop attacks

Epilepsy

Epilepsy is the syncope mimic that most physicians concern themselves with when faced with a victim of collapse (**Table 2**). In particular, because patients with syncope often show jerky movements of the arms and legs for a brief period, it is common that nonexpert bystanders report that the patient had a seizure. However, the jerky movements during syncope differ from those accompanying a grand mal epileptic seizure:

1. Are briefer in patients with syncope
2. Occur after the loss of consciousness has set in
3. Do not have the usual symmetric tonic-clonic features of a grand mal epileptic seizure

Psychogenic pseudosyncope (pseudoseizures)

Psychogenic pseudosyncope (often also termed psychogenic pseudoseizures) is the next most important syncope mimic.[68,91] The diagnosis relies on careful exclusion of other causes of syncope.

Table 2
Clinical features: syncope versus epilepsy

Clinical Findings	Seizure	Syncope
Eye-witness observations	Tonic-clonic movements coincide with loss of consciousness	Jerky movements start after loss of consciousness
	Relatively prolonged duration	Brief duration
	Automatisms such as chewing or lip-smacking are common	None
Symptoms before the event	Blue face	Nausea, vomiting, abdominal discomfort, hot/cold sensation
	Aura (such as unusual smell)	Discomfort, feeling of cold
	Pins and needles	Sweating (neurally mediated)
Postepisode symptoms	Prolonged confusion	Fatigue of variable duration

Tilt-table study may be useful to show an apparent faint in the absence of hemodynamic abnormality. In psychogenic pseudosyncope, there is no change in blood pressure or heart rate. An ILR may facilitate exclusion of arrhythmias in some cases.

Psychogenic pseudosyncope is often characterized by a greater frequency of symptoms than is expected for a true fainter (often multiple episodes in a day). A past history of sexual or physical abuse is often elicited in these patients. Psychiatric assessment is essential.

Other conditions

Other syncope mimics that need consideration but that are rarer include cataplexy (loss of muscle tone, often associated with a labile emotional personality), hyperventilation syndrome (syncope is unusual, whereas lightheadedness and a tingling sensation of the fingers or toes is more typical), and drop attacks.[92] The latter condition refers to a phenomenon in which there is a sudden fall without any apparent or recollected warning. Usually the events are too brief for patients to be certain whether there was any loss of consciousness. It is likely that many instances are caused by near-syncope or brief true syncope of conventional cases, particularly orthostatic hypotension.

SUMMARY

Syncope is a syndrome that is a particularly frequent cause for presentation to EDs and urgent-care clinics. The physician's key tasks are to establish a confident causal diagnosis, assess prognostic implications, and then provide appropriate advice to prevent recurrences. To achieve these goals, it is important to develop an organized approach to the assessment of the patient with syncope, the nature of which includes a careful initial examination as well as application of specialized syncope evaluation units and structured questionnaires for history taking. The initial patient evaluation, particularly a detailed medical history, is the key to identifying the most likely diagnosis. Based on findings from this initial step, subsequent carefully selected diagnostic tests can be chosen to confirm the clinical suspicion.

REFERENCES

1. Moya A, Sutton R, Ammirati F, et al, Task Force for the Diagnosis and Management of Syncope, European Society of Cardiology (ESC), European Heart Rhythm Association (EHRA), Heart Failure Association (HFA), Heart Rhythm Society (HRS). For the diagnosis and management of syncope (version 2009). Eur Heart J 2009;30(21):2631–71.
2. Blanc JJ, Benditt DG. Syncope: definition, classification, and multiple potential causes. In: Benditt DG, Blanc JJ, Brignole M, et al, editors. The evaluation and treatment of syncope. A handbook for clinical practice. Elmsford (NY): Futura Blackwell; 2003. p. 3–10.
3. Van Dijk JG, Thijs RD, Benditt DG, et al. A guide to disorders causing transient loss of consciousness: focus on syncope. Nat Rev Neurol 2009;5:438–48.
4. Kapoor WN. Evaluation and outcome of patients with syncope. Medicine (Baltimore) 1990;69:160–75.
5. Sun BC, Emond JA, Camargo CA Jr. Direct medical costs of syncope-related hospitalizations in the United States. Am J Cardiol 2005;95:668–71.
6. Baron-Esquivias G, Moreno SG, Martinez A, et al. Cost of diagnosis and treatment in patients admitted to a cardiology unit. Europace 2006;8:122–7.
7. Daccarett M, Jetter TL, Wasmund SL, et al. Syncope in the emergency department: comparison of standardized admission criteria with clinical practice. Europace 2011;13:1632–8.
8. Brignole M, Hamdan M. A standardized guideline-based algorithm coupled with online decision-making tool: the new frontier for efficient management of syncope? Europace 2011;13:1359–61.
9. Benditt DG, Can I. Initial evaluation of 'syncope and collapse': the need for a risk stratification consensus. J Am Coll Cardiol 2010;55:722–4.
10. Sheldon RS, Morillo CA, Krahn AD, et al. Standardized approaches to the investigation of syncope: Canadian Cardiovascular Society position paper. Can J Cardiol 2011;27:246–53.
11. Linzer M, Yang EH, Estes NA 3rd, et al. Diagnosing syncope. Part 1: value of history, physical examination, and electrocardiography. Ann Intern Med 1997; 126:989–96.
12. Rose MS, Koshman ML, Spreng S, et al. The relationship between health-related quality of life and frequency of spells in patients with syncope. J Clin Epidemiol 2000;53(12):1209–16.
13. Disertori M, Brignole M, Menozzi C, et al. Management of patients with syncope referred urgently to general hospitals. Europace 2003;5:283–91.
14. Blanc JJ, L'Her C, Touiza A, et al. Prospective evaluation and outcome of patients admitted for syncope over a 1 year period. Eur Heart J 2002; 23:815–20.
15. Gendelman HE, Linzer M, Gabelman M, et al. Syncope in a general hospital population. N Y State J Med 1983;83:116–65.
16. Wayne HH. Syncope: physiological considerations and an analysis of the clinical characteristics in 510 patients. Am J Med 1961;30:418–38.
17. Brignole M, Menozzi C, Bartoletti A, et al, For the Evaluation of Guidelines in Syncope Study 2 (EGSYS-2) group. A new management of syncope: prospective

guideline-based evaluation of patients referred urgently to general hospitals. Eur Heart J 2006;27: 76–82.

18. Savage DD, Corwin L, McGee DL, et al. Epidemiologic features of isolated syncope: the Framingham study. Stroke 1985;16:626–9.

19. Soteriades ES, Evans JC, Larson MG, et al. Incidence and prognosis of syncope. N Engl J Med 2002;347:878–85.

20. Chen LY, Shen WK, Mahoney DW, et al. Prevalence of syncope in a population aged more than 45 years. Am J Med 2006;119:1088.e1–7.

21. Sheldon RS, Serletis A. Epidemiological aspects of transient loss of consciousness/syncope. In: Benditt DG, Brignole M, Raviele A, et al, editors. Syncope and transient loss of consciousness. a multidisciplinary approach. Oxford (United Kingdom): Blackwell; 2007. p. 8–14.

22. Ganzeboom KS, Colman N, Reitsma JB, et al. Prevalence and triggers of syncope in medical students. Am J Cardiol 2003;91:1006–8.

23. Serletis A, Rose S, Sheldon AG, et al. Vasovagal syncope in medical students and their first-degree relatives. Eur Heart J 2006;27:1965–70.

24. Dermkesian G, Lamb LE. Syncope in a population of healthy young adults. J Am Med Assoc 1958;168: 1200–7.

25. Ungar A, Del Rosso A, Giada F, et al. Early and late outcome of treated patients referred for syncope to emergency department: the EGSYS2 follow-up study. Eur Heart J 2010;31:2021–6.

26. Sauer A, Moss A, McNitt S, et al. Long QT syndrome in adults. J Am Coll Cardiol 2007;49:329–52.

27. Paparella G, Sarkozy A, Brugada P. Brugada syndrome: the prognostic dilemma and value of syncope. Minerva Med 2009;100:307–19.

28. Ungar A, Mussi C, Del Rosso A, et al. Study of Syncope for the Italian Group for the Study of Syncope in the Elderly. Diagnosis and characteristics of syncope in older patients referred to geriatric departments. J Am Geriatr Soc 2006;54:1531–6.

29. Anpalahan M, Gibson S. Prevalence of neurally mediated syncope in older patients presenting with unexplained falls. Eur J Intern Med 2012;23(2): e48–52.

30. Kapoor WN, Peterson J, Wieand HS, et al. Diagnostic and prognostic implications of recurrences in patients with syncope. Am J Med 1987;83(4): 700–8.

31. Shen W, Decker W, Smars P, et al. Syncope evaluation in the emergency department study (SEEDS). A multidisciplinary approach to syncope management. Circulation 2004;110:3636–45.

32. Quinn J, McDermott D, Stiell I, et al. Prospective validation of the San Francisco syncope rule to predict patients with serious outcomes. Ann Emerg Med 2006;47:448–54.

33. Sun BC, Mangione CM, Merchant G. External validation of the San Francisco syncope rule. Ann Emerg Med 2007;49:420–7.

34. Colman N, Nahm K, van Dijk JG, et al. Diagnostic value of history taking in reflex syncope. Clin Auton Res 2004;14(Suppl 1):37–44.

35. Reed MJ, Newby DE, Coull AJ, et al. The ROSE (risk stratification of syncope in the emergency department) study. J Am Coll Cardiol 2010;55:713–21.

36. Costantino G, Perego F, Dipaola F, et al. Short- and long-term prognosis of syncope, risk factors, and role of hospital admission: results from the STePS (Short-Term Prognosis of Syncope) study. J Am Coll Cardiol 2008;51:276–83.

37. Grossman SA, Fischer C, Lipsitz LA, et al. Predicting adverse outcomes in syncope. J Emerg Med 2007; 33:233–9.

38. Colivicchi F, Ammirati F, Merlina D, et al, OESIL (Osservatorio Epidemiologico sulla Sincope nel Lazio) Study Investigators. Development and prospective validation of a risk stratification system for patients with syncope in the emergency department: the OESIL risk score. Eur Heart J 2003;24:811–9.

39. Sumner GL, Rose MS, Koshman ML, et al. Prevention of syncope trial recent history of vasovagal syncope in a young, referral-based population is a stronger predictor of recurrent syncope than lifetime syncope burden. J Cardiovasc Electrophysiol 2010;12:1375–80.

40. Alboni P, Brignole M, Menozzi C, et al. The diagnostic value of history in patients with syncope with or without heart disease. J Am Coll Cardiol 2001;37:1921–8.

41. Sarasin FP, Louis-Simonet M, Carballo D, et al. Prospective evaluation of patients with syncope: a population-based study. Am J Med 2001;111:177–84.

42. Oh JH, Hanusa BH, Kapoor WN. Do symptoms predict cardiac arrhythmias and mortality in patients with syncope. Arch Intern Med 1999;159:375–80.

43. Sheldon R, Rose S, Ritchie D, et al. Historical criteria that distinguish syncope from seizures. J Am Coll Cardiol 2002;40:142–8.

44. Romme JJ, van Dijk N, Boer R, et al. Diagnosing vasovagal syncope based on quantitative history taking: validation of the Calgary Syncope Score. Eur Heart J 2009;30:2888–96.

45. Del Rosso A, Ungar A, Maggi R, et al. Clinical predictors of cardiac syncope at initial evaluation in patients referred urgently to a general hospital: the EGSYS score. Heart 2008;94:1620–6.

46. Brignole M, Ungar A, Casagranda I, et al. Prospective multicentre systematic guideline-based management of patients referred to the syncope units of general hospitals. Europace 2010;12:109–18.

47. Benezet-Mazuecos J, Ibanez B, Rubio JM, et al. Utility of in-hospital cardiac remote telemetry in patients with unexplained syncope. Europace 2007; 9:1196–201.

48. Benditt DG, Samniah N, Pham S, et al. Effect of cough on heart rate and blood pressure in patients with "cough syncope". Heart Rhythm 2005;2:807–13.

49. Krediet CT, Parry SW, Jardine DL, et al. The history of diagnosing carotid sinus hypersensitivity: why are the current criteria too sensitive? Europace 2011;13:14–22.

50. Kenny RA, Ingram A, Bayliss J, et al. Head-up tilt: a useful test for investigating unexplained syncope. Lancet 1986;1:1352–5.

51. Benditt DG, Ferguson DW, Grubb BP, et al. Tilt table testing for assessing syncope. J Am Coll Cardiol 1996;28:263–75.

52. Morillo CA, Klein GJ, Zandri S, et al. Diagnostic accuracy of a low-dose isoproterenol head-up tilt protocol. Am Heart J 1995;129:901–6.

53. Bartoletti A, Alboni P, Ammirati F, et al. 'The Italian Protocol': a simplified head-up tilt testing potentiated with oral nitroglycerin to assess patients with unexplained syncope. Europace 2000;2:339–42.

54. Parry SW, Gray JC, Baptist M, et al. 'Front-loaded' glyceryl trinitrate-head-up tilt table testing: validation of a rapid first line tilt protocol for the diagnosis of vasovagal syncope. Age Ageing 2008;37:411–5.

55. Flammang D, Church T, Waynberger M, et al. Can adenosine 5'-triphosphate be used to select treatment in severe vasovagal syndrome? Circulation 1997;96:1201–8.

56. Perennes A, Fatemi M, Borel ML, et al. Epidemiology, clinical features, and follow-up of patients with syncope and a positive adenosine triphosphate test. J Am Coll Cardiol 2006;47:594–7.

57. Flammang D, Church TR, Roy LD, et al. Treatment of unexplained syncope: a multicenter randomized trial of cardiac pacing guided by adenosine 5'-triphosphate testing. Circulation 2012;235:31–6.

58. Benditt DG, Nguyen JT. Syncope: therapeutic approaches. J Am Coll Cardiol 2009;53:1741–51.

59. Samniah N, Sakaguchi S, Lurie KG, et al. Efficacy and safety of midodrine hydrochloride in patients with refractory vasovagal syncope. Am J Cardiol 2001;88:A80–3.

60. Perez-Lugones A, Schweikert R, Pavia S, et al. Usefulness of midodrine in patients with severely symptomatic neurocardiogenic syncope: a randomized control study. J Cardiovasc Electrophysiol 2001;12:935–8.

61. Romme JJ, van Dijk N, Go-Schon IK, et al. Effectiveness of midodrine in patients with recurrent vasovagal syncope not responding to non-pharmacological treatment (STAND-trial). Europace 2011;13:1639–47.

62. Brignole M, Sutton R, Menozzi C, et al. Early application of an implantable loop recorder allows effective specific therapy in patients with recurrent suspected neurally mediated syncope. Eur Heart J 2006;27:1085–92.

63. Brignole M, Menozzi C, Moya A, et al. Pacemaker therapy in patients with neutrally-mediated syncope

and asystole: Third International Study on Syncope of Uncertain Etiology (ISSUE-3): a randomized trial. Circulation 2012;125:2566–71.

64. Puggioni E, Guiducci V, Brignole M, et al. Results and complications of the carotid sinus massage performed according to the 'methods of symptoms'. Am J Cardiol 2002;89:599–601.

65. Tea SH, Mansourati J, L'Heveder G, et al. New insights into the pathophysiology of carotid sinus syndrome. Circulation 1996;93:1411–6.

66. Kerr SR, Pearce MS, Brayne C, et al. Carotid sinus hypersensitivity in asymptomatic older persons: implications for diagnosis of syncope and falls. Arch Intern Med 2006;166:515–20.

67. Davies AG, Kenny RA. Frequency of neurologic complications following carotid sinus massage. Am J Cardiol 1998;81:1256–7.

68. Sutton R, Brignole M, Benditt DG. Syncope. A focused review of key current management challenges. Nat Cardiol, in press.

69. Almquist A, Gornick CC, Benson DW Jr, et al. Carotid sinus hypersensitivity: evaluation of the vasodepressor component. Circulation 1985;71:927–37.

70. Smit AA, Halliwill JR, Low PA, et al. Pathophysiological basis of orthostatic hypotension in autonomic failure. J Physiol 1999;519:1–10.

71. Freeman R, Wieling W, Axelrod FB, et al. Consensus statement on definition of orthostatic hypotension, neurally mediated syncope and the postural tachycardia syndrome. Auton Neurosci 2011;161:46–8.

72. Freeman R, Wieling W, Axelrod FB, et al. Consensus statement on definition of orthostatic hypotension, neurally mediated syncope and the postural tachycardia syndrome. Clin Auton Res 2011;21:69–72.

73. Younoszai AK, Franklin WH, Chan DP, et al. Oral fluid therapy. A promising treatment for vasodepressor syncope. Arch Pediatr Adolesc Med 1998;152:165–8.

74. Lü F, Bergfeldt L. Role of electrophysiological testing in the evaluation of syncope. In: Benditt DG, Blanc JJ, Brignole M, et al, editors. The evaluation and treatment of syncope. A handbook for clinical practice. Elmsford (NY): Futura Blackwell; 2003. p. 80–95.

75. Moya A, Garcia-Civera R, Croci F, et al. Bradycardia detection in Bundle Branch Block (B4) study. Diagnosis, management, and outcomes of patients with syncope and bundle branch block. Eur Heart J 2011;32:1535–41.

76. Kulakowski P, Lelonek M, Krynski T, et al. Prospective evaluation of diagnostic work-up in syncope patients: results of the PL-US registry. Europace 2010;12:230–9.

77. Sarkozy A, Boussy T, Kourgiannides G, et al. Long-term follow-up of primary prophylactic implantable cardioverter-defibrillator therapy in Brugada syndrome. Eur Heart J 2007;28:334–44.

78. Paul M, Gerss J, Schulze-Bahr E, et al. Role of programmed ventricular stimulation in patients with

Brugada syndrome: a meta-analysis of worldwide published data. Eur Heart J 2007;28:2126–33.

79. Olshansky B, Hahn EA, Hartz VL, et al. Clinical significance of syncope in the electrophysiologic study versus electrocardiographic monitoring (ESVEM) trial. The ESVEM investigators. Am Heart J 1999; 137(5):878–86.

80. Steinberg JS, Beckman K, Greene HL, et al. Follow-up of patients with unexplained syncope and inducible ventricular tachyarrhythmias: analysis of the AVID registry and an AVID substudy. Antiarrhythmics versus implantable defibrillators. J Cardiovasc Electrophysiol 2001;12(9):996–1001.

81. Knight BP, Goyal R, Pelosi F, et al. Outcome of patients with nonischemic dilated cardiomyopathy and unexplained syncope treated with an implantable defibrillator. J Am Coll Cardiol 1999;33:1964–70.

82. Olshansky B, Poole JE, Johnson G, et al. Syncope predicts the outcome of cardiomyopathy patients: analysis of the SCD-HeFT study. J Am Coll Cardiol 2008;51:1277–85.

83. Prasad K, Williams L, Campbell R, et al. Syncope in hypertrophic cardiomyopathy: evidence for inappropriate vasodilation. Heart 2008;94:1312–7.

84. Kulbertus HE. Ventricular arrhythmias, syncope and sudden death in aortic stenosis. Eur Heart J 1988; 9(Suppl E):51–2.

85. Pires LA, May LM, Ravi S, et al. Comparison of event rates and survival in patients with unexplained syncope without documented ventricular tachyarrhythmias versus patients with documented sustained ventricular tachyarrhythmias both treated with implantable cardioverter-defibrillators. Am J Cardiol 2000;85:725–8.

86. Napolitano C, Bloise R, Monteforte N, et al. Sudden cardiac death and genetic ion channelopathies: long QT, Brugada, short QT, catecholaminergic polymorphic ventricular tachycardia, and idiopathic ventricular fibrillation. Circulation 2012;125:2027–32.

87. Carabello BA, Paulus WJ. Aortic stenosis. Lancet 2009;373:956–66.

88. Aronow WS. Recognition and management of aortic stenosis in the elderly. Geriatrics 2007;62:23–32.

89. Spirito P, Autore C, Rapezzi C, et al. Syncope and risk of sudden death in hypertrophic cardiomyopathy. Circulation 2009;119(13):1703–10.

90. Williams L, Frenneaux M. Syncope in hypertrophic cardiomyopathy and consequences for treatment. Europace 2007;9:817–22.

91. Benbadis SR, Chichkova R. Psychogenic pseudosyncope: an underestimated and provable diagnosis. Epilepsy Behav 2006;9:106–10.

92. Thijs RD, Bloem BR, van Dijk JG. Falls, faints, fits, and funny turns. J Neurol 2009;256:155–67.

Syncope Risk Stratification in the Emergency Department

Giorgio Costantino, MD[a],*, Raffaello Furlan, MD[b]

KEYWORDS

- Syncope • T-LoC • Risk stratification • Rule • Score • Emergency department

KEY POINTS

- Identify syncope through a detailed history (whenever this is not feasible, any presumed transient loss of consciousness should be considered and managed as syncope).
- Rule out syncope causes that may lead to a rapid clinical deterioration.
- Stratify patients according to risk (clinical judgment, a risk score, or a rule can be used). It is advisable to use the proposed criteria rather than a single anecdotal rule or risk score.
- Use monitoring procedures before deciding on hospitalization.
- Restrict the use of biomarkers to limited and specific cases.

CASE HISTORY

An 89-year-old woman was seen at the emergency department (ED) complaining of a transient loss of consciousness. Her daughter reported that she suddenly felt as though she were going to die and then suddenly passed out; consciousness was regained after what was described as an endless time, whereas weakness, lightheadedness, and nausea endured for several hours. No additional symptoms, including chest pain and dyspnea, were reported. Physical examination was normal apart from a known cardiac systolic murmur. The electrocardiogram (ECG) confirmed a previously known atrial fibrillation with a ventricular rate of 80 beats per minute. Blood pressure was 130/80 mm Hg. Laboratory tests were within the normal range. Her past history was characterized by arterial hypertension, depression, and a stroke, with the stroke resulting in some memory deficit. She was on warfarin, enalapril, and citalopram.

During the previous 2 weeks, she had been to the ED twice. The first time she was evaluated because of a near syncope while seating after dinner and, 1 week later, a sudden episode with near-syncope symptoms prompted her to go the ED. On both occasions, after a brief observation, she was discharged from the ED with a diagnosis of anxiety.

What steps should be taken to deal with a patient presenting at the ED because of a transient loss of consciousness?

THE FIRST STEP: IDENTIFYING PATIENTS WITH SYNCOPE

To identify the patient with syncope, 3 major issues have to be addressed:

- Distinguish patients with syncope from those with a transient loss of consciousness (T-LoC) of nonsyncopal origin
- Differentiate patients with syncope from those having falls
- Determine how to manage patients presenting with near syncope

---

The authors have nothing to disclose.
[a] Unità Operativa di Medicina Interna II, Dipartimento di Scienze Cliniche "L. Sacco," Ospedale L. Sacco, Università degli Studi di Milano, Via GB Grassi 74, Milano 20157, Italy; [b] Unità Operativa di Clinica Medica, Humanitas Clinical and Research Center, Università degli Studi di Milano, Via Manzoni 56, Rozzano 20089, Milan, Italy
* Corresponding author.
E-mail address: giorgic@libero.it

Cardiol Clin 31 (2013) 27–38
http://dx.doi.org/10.1016/j.ccl.2012.10.003
0733-8651/13/$ – see front matter © 2013 Elsevier Inc. All rights reserved.

Distinguish Patients with Syncope from Those with a T-LoC of Nonsyncopal Origin

Syncope is defined by the European Society of Cardiology (ESC) guidelines as a T-LoC caused by transient global cerebral hypoperfusion characterized by rapid onset, short duration, and spontaneous complete recovery.[1] Therefore, syncope must be differentiated from those situations in which T-LoC is not induced by a global cerebral hypoperfusion, as it is in the case of epilepsy, hypoglycemia, stroke, and carbon monoxide intoxication.

This pathophysiologic definition is important for diagnostic and therapeutic purposes, but it is of limited use in daily clinical practice because cerebral blood flow cannot be quantified during syncope in every patient. Moreover, until a definitive diagnosis is made, it is impossible to identify the pathophysiologic mechanism underlying an undetermined syncope, which accounts for up to 40% of all events.[1,2]

In keeping with a recent consensus study by Sun and colleagues,[3] we suggest a practical approach that defines as syncope all T-LoC of presumptive syncopal origin.

Differentiate Patients with Syncope from Those Having Falls

In clinical practice, it is often impossible to differentiate syncope and falls. Consider the case of an 82-year-old woman who lives alone and is found in the morning by her son on the floor, having likely been there since the evening before. Given that patients are seldom aware of their transient loss of consciousness, in the absence of a witness there is no way to discriminate between a loss of consciousness caused by syncope and one induced by a fall. This concept highlights the crucial role played by a careful history taken from a witness in facilitating the diagnosis during the early evaluation in the ED.

In keeping with these considerations, whenever it is impossible to discriminate between syncope and fall, any T-LoC should initially be considered and managed as syncope, because of its potential adverse outcome. Thereafter the patient should enter the risk stratification process followed by a careful cost benefits evaluation. This latter must always be done before any therapeutic option is started, particularly when potential significant side effects may take place, such as in the case of pacemaker or implantable cardioverter-defibrillator (ICD) implants.

Determine how to Manage Patients Presenting with Near Syncope (Presyncope)

At present, the management of patients with presyncope is largely heterogeneous worldwide.[3,4]

Presyncope (or near syncope) refers to the feeling of impending LoC without losing consciousness. Several symptoms and physical signs contribute to this subjective feeling, including weakness, lightheadedness, tunnel vision, dizziness, nausea, sweating, and pallor.

Because near syncope can be an indistinct condition and because it is often assumed that its prognosis is better than that of syncope, many studies on syncope performed in the ED excluded patients with presyncope at enrollment.[5–7] In contrast, other investigators[8] assumed that syncope and near syncope were identical. To answer this question, Grossman and colleagues[4] compared the clinical outcome of patients with presyncope with that of individuals with syncope and found no difference. The investigators concluded that the prognosis of near syncope was similar to that of syncope, but this statement has been questioned[9–11] and data are not available from which to draw definitive conclusions.

Based on these considerations and on the lack of evidence, a physician should judge case by case whether a presyncope episode ought to be considered as a syncope.

It cannot directly be concluded that the 89-year-old patient discussed earlier has syncope (according to the ESC definition, a T-LoC caused by a global cerebral hypoperfusion). That episode can be considered a T-LoC of presumptive syncopal origin, and the patient's past history had no diabetes or epilepsy to suggest a T-LoC of nonsyncopal origin. She did not fall, because the daughter ruled out this possibility. In addition, in our opinion, in the presence of risk factors (age, sudden syncope without preliminary symptoms, abnormal ECG), the 2 previous presyncope episodes should be regarded as syncope.

THE SECOND STEP: RULING OUT CAUSES OF SYNCOPE THAT MAY LEAD TO A RAPID CLINICAL DETERIORATION

The overall risk for a patient entering the ED because of syncope is between 5% and 15%, and the mortality at 1 week is about 1%.[5,7,8,10,11] The primary goal of the ED physician is thus to discriminate individuals at low risk who can be safely discharged, from patients at high risk who require prompt hospitalization for monitoring and/or appropriate treatment.

Once a subject has been identified as having had syncope, the diseases potentially leading to a rapid clinical deterioration should be ruled out (**Box 1**). See the articles as discussed by Krahn and colleagues elsewhere in this issue.

THE THIRD STEP: STRATIFYING THE PATIENT WITH SYNCOPE ACCORDING TO RISK

Undetermined syncope is common after the first assessment in the ED. Thus, in the absence of a positive diagnosis, the doctor's main goal should shift from the effort to further identify a syncope

---

Box 1
Potential life-threatening disorders leading to syncope

Cardiovascular

Arrhythmias

- Ventricular tachycardia
- Bradycardia: Mobitz type II or third-degree heart block
- Significant sinus pause (>3 seconds)

ECG features that can suggest an arrhythmic origin

- Long QT syndrome
- Brugada syndrome

Ischemia

- Acute coronary syndrome, myocardial infarction

Structural abnormalities

- Valvular heart disease: aortic stenosis, mitral stenosis
- Cardiomyopathy (ischemic, dilated, hypertrophic)
- Atrial myxoma
- Cardiac tamponade
- Aortic dissection

Significant hemorrhage

- Trauma with significant blood loss
- Gastrointestinal bleeding
- Tissue rupture: aortic aneurysm, spleen, ovarian cyst, ectopic pregnancy
- Retroperitoneal hemorrhage

Pulmonary embolism

- Saddle embolus resulting in outflow tract obstruction or severe hypoxia

Subarachnoid hemorrhage

---

cause to an attempt to stratify the patient risk. This stratification can be done from the patient's history and the characteristics of the syncope. Risk stratification can be obtained from clinical experience (clinical judgment) or by using appropriate rules or risk scores. Rules or risk scores may help the ED physician in decision making, although so far there is no compelling evidence that any score or rule performs better than personal clinical judgment in affecting patients' clinical outcomes.[10–14]

Rules

Rules were developed to stratify the risks of a single patient presenting for syncope in the ED. Most rules were obtained and derived in the ED setting and are intended to assess short-term outcomes. Rules encompass the presence or absence of different dichotomous variables as risk factors. If a single variable is present, then the patient is stratified as high risk and requiring hospital admission.

Examples of such rules are the risk stratification of syncope in the emergency department (Rose), San Francisco Syncope Rule (SFSR), and Boston Syncope Rules,[7,8,15] with the SFSR[8] being the only rules that are externally validated.

SFSR

The SFSR was first published in 2004 by Quinn and colleagues[8] based on 684 subjects seen for syncope or near syncope in the ED. The investigators found that the presence of any of the variables summarized in **Table 1** had a sensitivity of 96% (95% confidence interval [CI] 92%–100%) and a specificity of 62% (95% CI 58%–66%) for predicting adverse events at 1-week follow-up. Death, myocardial infarction, arrhythmia, pulmonary embolism, stroke, subarachnoid hemorrhage, significant hemorrhage, or any condition causing or likely to cause a new clinical evaluation at ED or a new hospitalization for a related event were considered adverse events. The SFSR has been validated by the same investigators in a separate cohort of 791 patients, obtaining a sensitivity of 98% (95% CI 89%–100%) and a specificity of 56% (95% CI 52%–60%) for adverse events at 30-day follow-up.[16] The use of this rule would have resulted in a 7% potential reduction of hospital admissions (**Tables 2** and **3**).

Since its first reports, the SFSR has been externally validated by other investigators, with discordant results.[10,17–19] These inconsistencies might be related to the heterogeneous ECG interpretation characterizing those studies.[10] For example, Quinn and colleagues[20,21] considered as an abnormal ECG any new alteration, including the

Table 1
Features of different syncope risk stratification tools

Rule/Score	Acronym	Variables	How Does It Work?
SFSR	CHESS	Congestive heart failure, history of: Hematocrit <30% ECG, abnormal Shortness of breath Systolic blood pressure at triage <90 mm Hg	Patient at high risk if a single variable is present
Rose	BRACES	BNP level ≥300 pg/mL or bradycardia ≤50 in ED or before hospital Rectal examination showing fecal occult blood (if suspicion of gastrointestinal bleeding) Anemia: hemoglobin ≤90 g/L Chest pain ECG showing Q wave (not in lead III) Saturation ≤94% on room air	Patient at high risk if a single variable is present
BOSTON[a]	None	I. Signs and symptoms of acute coronary syndrome II. Worrisome cardiac history III. Family history of sudden death IV. Valvular heart disease V. Signs of conduction disease VI. Volume depletion VII. Persistent (>15 min) abnormal vital signs in the ED without the need for concurrent intervention such as oxygen, pressor drugs, temporary pacemakers VIII. CNS	Patient at high risk if a single variable is present
OESIL	None	History of cardiovascular disease Abnormal ECG Age >65 y Absence of prodromal symptoms	Single factor counts as 1. Sum ≤1 = low risk; sum >1 = high risk
EGSYS	None	Palpitations preceding syncope (4 pts) Heart disease, abnormal ECG, or both (3 pts) Syncope during effort (3 pts) Syncope while supine (2 pts) Precipitating or predisposing factors, or both (warm, crowded place/prolonged orthostasis/fear-pain-emotion) (−1 pts) Autonomic prodromes (nausea/vomiting) (−1 pts)	Score ≥3 pts is considered positive

Abbreviations: BNP, brain natriuretic peptide; EGSYS, Evaluation of Guidelines in Syncope Study; pts, points; OESIL, Osservatorio Epidemiologico sulla Sincope del Lazio; ROSE, Risk Stratification of Syncope in the Emergency Department; SFSR, San Francisco Syncope Rule.

[a] I: 1, complaint of chest pain of possible cardiac origin; 2, ischemic ECG changes (ST increase or deep [>0.1 mV] ST depression); 3, other ECG changes (VT, VF, supraventricular tachycardia [SVT], rapid atrial fibrillation, or new [or not known to be old] ST-T wave changes); 4, complaint of shortness of breath. II: 5, history of coronary artery disease, including deep Q waves and hypertrophic or dilated cardiomyopathy; 6, history of congestive heart failure or left ventricular dysfunction; 7, history of or current ventricular tachycardia, ventricular fibrillation; 8, history of pacemaker; 9, history of ICD; 10, prehospital use of antidysrhythmic medication excluding β-blockers or calcium channel blockers. III: 11, family history (first-degree relative) with sudden death, HOCM, Brugada syndrome, or long QT syndrome. IV: 12, heart murmur noted in history or on ED examination. V: 13, multiple syncopal episodes within the last 6 months; 14, rapid heart beat by patient history; 15, syncope during exercise; 16, QT interval >500 ms; 17, second-degree or third-degree heart block or intraventricular block. VI: 18, gastrointestinal bleeding by Hemoccult or history; 19, hematocrit <30; 20, dehydration not corrected in the ED per treating physician discretion. VII: 21, respiratory rate >24 breaths/min; 22, O₂ saturation <90%; 23, sinus rate <50 beats/min or sinus rate >100 beats/min; 24, blood pressure <90 mm Hg. VIII: 25, primary CNS event (ie, SAH, stroke).

Table 2
Features of the studies leading to a risk stratification tool and its external validation

Rule/ Score	Derivation Population	Validation Population	Setting; Follow-up	External Validation
SFSR	684 syncope or near syncope	791 patients with syncope or near syncope	ED; derivation 7 d, validation 30 d	Systematic review: sensitivity 87% (95% CI 79–93), and specificity of 52% (95% CI 43–62)[10]
Rose	550 patients	550 patients	ED; 30 d	None
BOSTON	None	362 patients	ED; 30 d	None
OESIL	270 patients in EDs, 1-y follow-up	328 patients, 1-y follow-up	ED; 1 y	Few studies[12]
EGSYS	260 patients	258 patients	ED; diagnosis of cardiac syncope on a predefined diagnostic item; mortality at 2 y	None

ECG abnormalities observed during a patient's monitoring in the ED. In contrast, other studies focused only on the ECG features obtained at ED presentation. Sacillotto and colleagues[10] assessed the sensitivity and specificity of that rule by a systematic review and reported a sensitivity of 87% (95% CI 79–93) and a specificity of 52% (95% CI 43–62). These investigators concluded that the SFSR can be useful in the decision-making process of admitting or discharging patients from the ED for those patients with undetermined syncope after ED evaluation. They concluded that a posttest probability of adverse events lower than 2% would be suitable to safely discharge patients. However, this conclusion is arbitrary because it does not take into account that the exclusion of the dangerous causes of syncope during the ED stay may reduce the likelihood of adverse events more than the reduction caused by a good performance of the rule. In addition, the SFSR did not provide clues to the clinical features of patients who should undergo continuous cardiovascular and respiratory monitoring.

The Rose rule

The Rose rule was published in 2010 and was derived and validated in a single ED center in Edimburgh.[7] Reed and colleagues[7] recruited 550 patients for deriving and 550 individuals for validating the rule and observed that the presence of at least 1 of the proposed variables (risk factors) had a sensitivity of 87% and a specificity of 66% for adverse events (see **Tables 1–3**). Adverse events included acute myocardial infarction, life-threatening arrhythmias (ventricular fibrillation,

sustained, ventricular tachycardia, ventricular pause >3 seconds), pacemaker or cardiac defibrillator implant within 1 month from the index syncope, pulmonary embolism, cerebrovascular accidents, intracranial or subarachnoid hemorrhage, hemorrhage requiring more than 2 units of blood transfusion, acute surgical procedures, or endoscopic intervention (see **Table 2**).

The limits of this rule are the poor sensitivity found during the internal validation and the need of a laboratory test (ie, B-type natriuretic peptides [BNP]). This latter limitation implies that all patients presenting in the ED for syncope should have bloods taken, thus partially diverging from the ESC syncope guideline suggestions[1] and everyday clinical practice. Moreover, no external validation of the rule is available at the moment.

The Boston Syncope Rule

The Boston Syncope Rule was first published in 2007 by Grossman and colleagues.[15] The investigators recruited 362 patients and considered the variables (risk factors) reported in the American College of Emergency Physicians' clinical policy on syncope.[22] Given the presence of at least 1 of the variables, the sensitivity and specificity of the rule was 97% (95% CI 93–100) and 62% (95% CI 56–69), respectively (see **Tables 1–3**).

Its complexity is the major weakness of this rule because more than 10 variables should be considered. In addition, some variables, such as primary central nervous system (CNS) events are adverse events themselves. This weakness does not help physician to decide which patient deserves closer observation, monitoring, or hospital admission,

Table 3
Adverse events and ECG features taken into account by the different risk stratification tools

Rule/Score	Anomalous ECG	Adverse Events
SFSR	Any new change In the absence of a previous ECG, any abnormality during ECG repetition or monitoring	Death, myocardial infarction, arrhythmias, pulmonary embolism, stroke, subarachnoid hemorrhage, significant hemorrhage, or any condition causing or likely to cause a return to ED and hospitalization for a related event
Rose	Q wave (not in lead III)	Acute myocardial infarction according to the universal definition, life-threatening arrhythmias (ventricular fibrillation, sustained ventricular tachycardia, ventricular pause >3 s), pacemaker or cardiac defibrillator implant within 1 mo of index collapse, pulmonary embolus, cerebrovascular accident, intracranial hemorrhage, or subarachnoid hemorrhage, hemorrhage requiring a blood transfusion of 2 units, acute surgical procedure, or endoscopic intervention
BOSTON	QT interval >500 ms Second-degree or third-degree heart block or intraventricular block Ischemic ECG changes (ST increase or ST depression [>0.1 mV]) Other ECG changes (VT, VF, SVT, rapid atrial fibrillation, or new [or not known to be old] ST), T wave changes, deep Q waves The sinus rate <50 beats/min or sinus rate >100 beats/min	Pacemaker/implantable cardiac defibrillator placement, percutaneous coronary intervention, surgery, blood transfusion, cardiopulmonary resuscitation, alterations in antidysrhythmic therapy, endoscopy with intervention, or correction of carotid stenosis, death, pulmonary embolus, stroke, severe infection/sepsis, ventricular dysrhythmia, atrial dysrhythmia (including SVT and atrial fibrillation with rapid ventricular response), intracranial bleed, hemorrhage, myocardial infarction, cardiac arrest, or life-threatening sequelae of syncope (ie, rhabdomyolysis, long bone or cervical spine fractures)
OESIL	Rhythm abnormalities (atrial fibrillation or flutter, SVT, multifocal atrial tachycardia, frequent or repetitive premature supraventricular or ventricular complexes, sustained or nonsustained ventricular tachycardia, paced rhythms) Atrioventricular or intraventricular conduction disorders (complete atrioventricular block, Mobitz I or Mobitz II atrioventricular block, bundle branch block or intraventricular conduction delay) Left or right ventricular hypertrophy; left axis deviation Old myocardial infarction, ST segment and T wave abnormalities consistent with or possibly related to myocardial ischemia	Death at follow-up

(continued on next page)

Table 3
(continued)

Rule/Score	Anomalous ECG	Adverse Events
Evaluation of Guidelines in Syncope Study (EGSYS)	Sinus bradycardia, atrioventricular block greater than first degree, bundle branch block Acute or old myocardial infarction Supraventricular or ventricular tachycardia Left or right ventricular hypertrophy, ventricular preexcitation long QT, and Brugada pattern	Diagnosis of cardiac syncope: Mechanical cardiac syncope (severe valvular stenosis, or other flow obstruction, acute myocardial ischemia) Arrhythmic syncope (sinus bradycardia, 40 beats/min or repetitive sinoatrial blocks or sinus pauses of 3 s; Mobitz 2 or advanced second-degree atrioventricular block or third-degree atrioventricular block; alternating left and right bundle branch block, pacemaker malfunction with cardiac pauses, rapid paroxysmal supraventricular or ventricular tachyarrhythmias) electrophysiologic study alterations

because in the presence of an acute cerebral hemorrhage it is self-evident that hospital admission is mandatory.

Scores

Although rules consider the presence of a specific variable sufficient to put the patient in a high-risk class, scores incorporate several variables. These variables are combined to derive a score that enables the prediction of the subsequent risk to the patient.

The scores were built up mostly by cardiologists and are typically aimed at identifying cardiac adverse events. This article discusses the Osservatorio Epidemiologico sulla Sincope del Lazio (OESIL) and the EGSYS risk scores.

OESIL risk score

OESIL was published in 2003[23] based on a derivation cohort in which Colivicchi and colleagues[23] recruited 270 patients presenting to ED for syncope. The validation cohort was subsequently based on 328 individuals. The data suggested that the presence of anomalous ECG, absence of presyncope symptoms, history of cardiovascular disease, and age older than 65 years were the risk factors associated with a poor prognosis at 1-year follow-up (see **Tables 1–3**). Later, the OESIL risk score was externally validated using the Short-Term Prognosis of Syncope (STePS)[5] population and compared with the SFSR by Dipaola and colleagues.[12] In the work by Dipaola and colleagues,[12] our group showed that the OESIL risk score had a sensitivity of 88% (95% CI

70–98) and a specificity of 60% (95% CI 55–64), and the SFSR 81% (95% CI 61–93) and 63% (95% CI 58–67), in predicting an adverse outcome within 10 days. The clinical judgment (ie, the doctor's decision to admit or discharge patients from ED independently of any strict adherence to predefined protocol or risk scores) had a sensitivity of 77% (95% CI 56–91) and a specificity of 69% (95% CI 64–73). The sensitivities of the 3 decision-making approaches were not significantly different, but the SFSR and OESIL would have recognized all 5 patients who died within 10 days from syncope, whereas the clinical judgment missed 2 deaths. However, the numbers of patients and events were inadequate to draw definitive conclusions. Although derived on events at 1 year, the OESIL risk score proved to be useful even in the short-term risk stratification of patients with syncope. Major limitations of OESIL result from the small number of its independent validations, whereas its main strength is its simplicity, which enables its use even by nurses triaging patients with syncope.

EGSYS score

The EGSYS score was derived and internally validated by Del Rosso and colleagues.[6] It is the only score that considered as events the different causes of syncope and it was specifically aimed at identifying a cardiac cause of the syncopal episode. The investigators reported that the score is characterized by a sensitivity of 92% (95% CI 77–98) and specificity of 69% (95% CI 63–75). There are no external validations of such a score, particularly in the emergency setting, and, for this reason, the score is likely to be more useful in a cardiologic setting than in the ED, where syncope episodes induced by noncardiac diseases are more frequent (see **Tables 1–3**).

Table 4 compares the strength and weakness of different rules and scores used for syncope risk stratification.

Let us try to stratify the risk after syncope of the 89-year-old patient discussed earlier, by using the previously mentioned clinical rules and risk scores.

The patient would have been stratified as being at significant risk, thus deserving hospital admission, according to the Rose rule (ECG positive), OESIL risk score (ECG, age), EGSYS score (ECG and cardiovascular history), and Boston (multiple syncope, cardiac systolic murmur). In contrast, at admission in the ED she would have been stratified as being at low risk according to the SFSR. However, her recurrence of syncope, age, and cardiovascular history would make any physician uncomfortable about an early discharge.

To make this evaluation easier for the reader, this article discusses the strengths and limitations of the different rules or risk scores in **Table 4**.

The hospitalization rates related to syncope vary widely worldwide, ranging from 15% to 65%.[2] This variation may be secondary to the differing organization of health care systems; to the consequent different patients' health care patterns; to the availability of both inpatient and outpatient facilities for prompt syncope diagnosis and therapy, such as those provided by a syncope unit[24]; and to physicians' personal knowledge of this disorder and awareness of guidelines and clinical risk scores.

A recent investigation[14] emphasized the lack of evidence that syncope decision rules might improve syncope diagnostic accuracy or reduce work-up costs, thus challenging their usefulness. A new tool for syncope management is represented by the syncope unit,[24] in which differing medical competence and several facilities are functionally combined, as discussed in a dedicated article elsewhere in this issue. **Fig. 1** shows a flow diagram of a possible syncope approach in the ED.

Do any of the risk rules or scores identify people who might have adverse outcomes caused by syncope, or do they simply identify people who will have an adverse outcome and happen to have syncope?

Based on our previous observations,[5] there are 2 clinically important time frames for syncope. The early period (hours and days) following syncope characterized by the largest mortality because of a new and still undiagnosed life-threatening disorder leading to syncope, and a second period characterized by a time scale of months or years in which comorbidity and frailty play a major role. Because there is a low rate of adverse events following syncope, the risk scores and clinical rules are likely to better identify frailty than patients' short-term risk, which might account for the poor performance of the rule/scores in identifying short-term adverse clinical outcomes.[10–12]

Based on these considerations, the role of clinical decision rules or risk scores and their comparison with clinical judgment in the management of patients presenting in the ED for syncope remain to be elucidated. In addressing syncope, risk scores and decision rules can be useful by highlighting the critical variables that should be considered and we expect that the international single-patient meta-analysis currently in progress will provide a tentative answer to these issues.

Table 4
Comparison of different rules/risk scores

Rule/Score	Strengths	Limitations
SFSR	User friendly Derived in the ED All adverse events considered Several external validations	Inconsistency in validations results Decision of patients monitoring at physician's discretion
Rose	User friendly Derived in the ED All adverse events considered	Need venous sample Not externally validated Limited sensitivity compared with other rules
BOSTON	Derived in the ED All adverse events considered	Complicated Overlap between risk factors and adverse events
OESIL	User friendly	Not derived in the ED
EGSYS	User friendly Considered cardiac cause of syncope	Not derived in the ED Not consider all adverse events

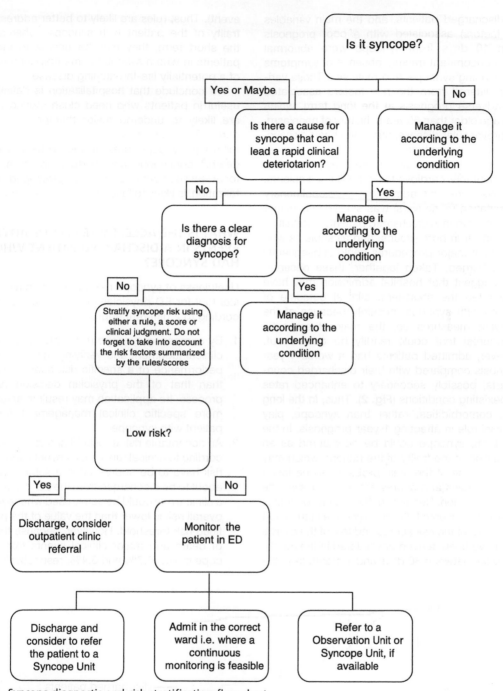

Fig. 1. Syncope diagnostic and risk stratification flow chart.

DOES HOSPITAL ADMISSION AFFECT SYNCOPE PROGNOSIS?

Difficulties in promptly addressing the cause of syncope in the emergency setting and concerns about fatal arrhythmias and sudden death often lead to an excessive hospital admission rate, with increasing costs.[2] For this reason, whether or not hospital admission significantly affects the outcome is an important issue.

The STePS study performed by our group specifically addressed this topic[5] and included 676 consecutive patients who presented for syncope in 4 EDs. Both short-term (ie, within 10 days) and long-term (ie, within 1 year) adverse events were assessed and compared in admitted and discharged patients, and the main variables (risk factors) associated with a poor prognosis within 10 days from syncope were abnormal ECG, concomitant trauma, absence of symptoms of impending syncope, and male sex. Those variables differed from the risk factors associated with adverse prognosis in the long term, which were age older than 65 years, history of neoplasm, cerebrovascular disease, structural heart disease, and ventricular arrhythmia. Although the number of major therapeutic procedures (ie, pacemaker or implantable cardioverter-defibrillator implants, intensive care unit admission, cardiopulmonary resuscitation maneuvers) was significantly higher in admitted than in discharged patients, mortalities were similar in both groups, and all subjects who underwent major procedures could subsequently be discharged. Taken together, these observations suggest that hospital admission may have ameliorated the short-term clinical outcome of patients with syncope, possibly because of the lifesaving measures (ie, the major therapeutic procedures) that could readily be carried out. However, admitted patients had a worse 1-year prognosis compared with their discharged counterparts, possibly secondary to enhanced rates of coexisting conditions (**Fig. 2**). Thus, in the long term, comorbidities, rather than syncope, play a crucial role in affecting 1-year prognosis. In the long term, syncope could be considered as an expression of the frailty of the patient, which may represent one of the main problems to be faced whenever rules and scores are used for syncope risk stratification. Because of the paucity of deaths and adverse events following syncope in the short term, most of the risk scores and few of the clinical rules have been derived or validated in the middle period (ie, between 30 days and 1 month from the

event). Thus, rules are likely to better address the frailty of the patient with syncope, whereas, in the short term, they may be unable to identify patients in whom syncope is the epiphenomenon of a potentially life-threatening disease.

We conclude that hospitalization is definitively useful in patients who need close monitoring or are likely to undergo major therapeutic procedures. Based on the observation that the 48 hours following syncope present the highest risk for death,[5] continuous cardiorespiratory monitoring for at least 48 hours, rather than a prolonged hospitalization, is likely to favorably affect the prognosis.

WHAT IS THE ACCEPTABLE RISK OF ADVERSE EVENTS IN A DISCHARGED PATIENT WHO HAD SYNCOPE?

Usefulness of syncope risk stratification as a clinical tool for ED physicians can be evaluated according to 2 different approaches:

1. By comparing syncope risk scales with simple clinical judgment and verifying that the overall performance of a specific risk score is higher than that of the physician decision-making process. Its application may result in safer and more specific clinical management for the patient with syncope.
2. An acceptable risk threshold has to be set. According to clinical rules, major events and death risk have to be addressed in a subject who is about to be discharged from the ED. Thereafter, a clinical rule could be safely used whenever the overall risk is lower than the value of the predefined risk threshold. However, because the risk of death and major clinical events from syncope is low (0.7% and 5.4%, respectively),[5] an

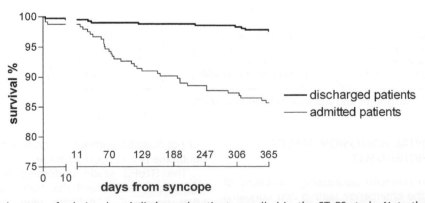

Fig. 2. Survival curves of admitted and discharged patients enrolled in the STePS study. Note that discharged patients had lower long-term mortality than admitted individuals. (*Modified from* Costantino G, Perego F, Dipaola F, et al. Short- and long-term prognosis of syncope, risk factors, and role of hospital admission: results from the STePS (Short-Term Prognosis of Syncope) study. J Am Coll Cardiol 2008;51:276–83; with permission.)

acceptable risk is hard to define. Moreover, there is no consensus about risk thresholds, and different groups consider different thresholds to be acceptable.[10,25]

ARE LABORATORY BIOMARKERS USEFUL FOR ED CLINICAL DECISION MAKING?

The European syncope guidelines do not consider routine tests, as assessed by a venous sample, to be appropriate for syncope evaluation in all patients.[1] However, D-dimer and other biomarkers have attracted interest for risk stratification in the ED.

D-Dimer

There is evidence that the routine measurement of D-dimer in patients presenting to the ED for syncope is useless both for identifying the cause of syncope and as a prognostic index.[26] D-dimer may have a significant role in selected syncope cases in which there is significant suspicion for pulmonary embolism or aortic dissection.[27]

Troponin

There is evidence that routine measurement of troponin is of limited effectiveness in the ED management of the patient with syncope, although it can be useful in selected cases in which acute coronary syndrome is suspected.[28] There are no conclusive data on the use of ultrasensitive troponin assays.

BNPs

N-Terminal pro–brain natriuretic peptide (NT-proBNP) and BNP have been used to assess the prognosis and cause of syncope. In the Rose decision rule,[7] the plasma BNP level was proposed as a reliable marker for syncope risk stratification. In addition, BNP was recommended to discriminate cardiac and noncardiac causes of syncope. Increased BNP and NT-proBNP plasma levels have been observed in arrhythmias and these peptides have thus raised interest as biomarkers of arrhythmic syncope.[29] Pfister and colleagues[30] suggested the use of NT-proBNP to differentiate arrhythmic from nonarrhythmic syncope. However, a single BNP assessment is largely influenced by comorbidities[31] and we reported[32] that the time course of BNP and NT-proBNP changes following an induced ventricular fibrillation had a peak of increase of both biomarkers 9 hours after the event. These data suggested that the use of BNP kinetics, rather than single plasma measurements, could be useful both to identify a potential arrhythmic cause of syncope and for patient risk stratification, but

prospective studies are expected to confirm this hypothesis.

The 89-year-old patient discussed earlier felt that she was going to die during ECG continuous monitoring in the ED. The ECG showed a 4-second pause. A permanent pacemaker was placed and, so far, the patient has not had another syncope spell.

ACKNOWLEDGMENTS

We would like to acknowledge all STePS investigators, and in particular Carlo Selmi, Franca Dipaola, Mattia Bonzi, and Ilaria Bossi, for their valuable comments and suggestions.

REFERENCES

1. Moya A, Sutton R, Ammirati F, et al. Guidelines for the diagnosis and management of syncope (version 2009). Eur Heart J 2009;30:2631–71.
2. D'Ascenzo F, Biondi-Zoccai G, Reed MJ, et al. Incidence, etiology and predictors of adverse outcomes in 43,315 patients presenting to the emergency department with syncope: an international meta-analysis. Int J Cardiol 2011. [Epub ahead of print].
3. Sun BC, Thiruganasambandamoorthy V, Cruz JD. Standardized reporting guidelines for emergency department syncope risk-stratification research. Acad Emerg Med 2012;19:694–702.
4. Grossman SA, Babineau M, Burke L, et al. Do outcomes of near syncope parallel syncope? Am J Emerg Med 2012;30:203–6.
5. Costantino G, Perego F, Dipaola F, et al. Short- and long-term prognosis of syncope, risk factors, and role of hospital admission: results from the STePS (Short-Term Prognosis of Syncope) study. J Am Coll Cardiol 2008;51:276–83.
6. Del Rosso A, Ungar A, Maggi R, et al. Clinical predictors of cardiac syncope at initial evaluation in patients referred urgently to a general hospital: the EGSYS score. Heart 2008;94:1620–6.
7. Reed MJ, Newby DE, Coull AJ, et al. The ROSE (Risk Stratification of Syncope in the Emergency Department) study. J Am Coll Cardiol 2010;55:713–21.
8. Quinn JV, Stiell IG, McDermott DA, et al. Derivation of the San Francisco Syncope Rule to predict patients with short-term serious outcomes. Ann Emerg Med 2004;43:224–32.
9. Cernuschi G, Bonzi M, Fiorelli E, et al. Do outcomes of near syncope parallel syncope? Am J Emerg Med 2012. [Epub ahead of print].
10. Saccilotto RT, Nickel CH, Bucher HC, et al. San Francisco Syncope Rule to predict short-term serious outcomes: a systematic review. CMAJ 2011;183:E1116–26.

11. Serrano LA, Hess EP, Bellolio MF, et al. Accuracy and quality of clinical decision rules for syncope in the emergency department: a systematic review and meta-analysis. Ann Emerg Med 2010; 56:362–73.

12. Dipaola F, Costantino G, Perego F, et al. San Francisco syncope rule, osservatorio epidemiologico sulla sincope nel lazio risk score, and clinical judgment in the assessment of short-term outcome of syncope. Am J Emerg Med 2010;28:432–9.

13. Perego F, Costantino G, Dipaola F, et al. Predictors of hospital admission after syncope: relationships with clinical risk scores. Int J Cardiol 2012. [Epub ahead of print].

14. Sheldon RS, Morillo CA, Krahn AD, et al. Standardized approaches to the investigation of syncope: Canadian Cardiovascular Society position paper. Can J Cardiol 2011;27:246–53.

15. Grossman SA, Fischer C, Lipsitz LA, et al. Predicting adverse outcomes in syncope. J Emerg Med 2007; 33:233–9.

16. Quinn J, McDermott D, Stiell I, et al. Prospective validation of the San Francisco Syncope Rule to predict patients with serious outcomes. Ann Emerg Med 2006;47:448–54.

17. Sun BC, Mangione CM, Merchant G, et al. External validation of the San Francisco Syncope Rule. Ann Emerg Med 2007;49:420–7.

18. Thiruganasambandamoorthy V, Hess EP, Alreesi A, et al. External validation of the San Francisco Syncope Rule in the Canadian setting. Ann Emerg Med 2010;55:464–72.

19. Birnbaum A, Esses D, Bijur P, et al. Failure to validate the San Francisco Syncope Rule in an independent emergency department population. Ann Emerg Med 2008;52:151–9.

20. Quinn J, McDermott D. ECG criteria of the San Francisco Syncope Rule. Ann Emerg Med 2011; 57:72–3.

21. Quinn J, McDermott D. Electrocardiogram findings in emergency department patients with syncope. Acad Emerg Med 2011;18:714–8.

22. American College of Emergency Physicians. Clinical policy: critical issues in the evaluation and management of patients presenting with syncope. Ann Emerg Med 2001;37:771–6.

23. Colivicchi F, Ammirati F, Melina D, et al. Development and prospective validation of a risk stratification system for patients with syncope in the emergency department: the OESIL risk score. Eur Heart J 2003; 24:811–9.

24. Shen WK, Decker WW, Smars PA, et al. Syncope Evaluation in the Emergency Department Study (SEEDS): a multidisciplinary approach to syncope management. Circulation 2004;110:3636–45.

25. McNally M, Curtain J, O'Brien KK, et al. Validity of British Thoracic Society guidance (the CRB-65 rule) for predicting the severity of pneumonia in general practice: systematic review and meta-analysis. Br J Gen Pract 2010;60:e423–33.

26. Stockley CJ, Reed MJ, Newby DE, et al. The utility of routine D-dimer measurement in syncope. Eur J Emerg Med 2009;16:256–60.

27. Dipaola F, Cucchi I, Filardo N, et al. Syncope as a symptom of non-massive pulmonary embolism: a case report. Intern Emerg Med 2006;1:167–70.

28. Reed MJ, Newby DE, Coull AJ, et al. Diagnostic and prognostic utility of troponin estimation in patients presenting with syncope: a prospective cohort study. Emerg Med J 2010;27:272–6.

29. Pfister R, Diedrichs H, Larbig R, et al. NT-pro-BNP for differential diagnosis in patients with syncope. Int J Cardiol 2009;133:51–4.

30. Pfister R, Hagemeister J, Esser S, et al. NT-pro-BNP for diagnostic and prognostic evaluation in patients hospitalized for syncope. Int J Cardiol 2012;155(2): 268–72.

31. Costantino G, Solbiati M, Pisano G, et al. NT-pro-BNP for differential diagnosis in patients with syncope. Int J Cardiol 2009;137:298–9.

32. Costantino G, Solbiati M, Sagone A, et al. Time course of B-type natriuretic peptides changes after ventricular fibrillation: relationships with cardiac syncope. Int J Cardiol 2011;153:333–5.

Syncope Units
Impact on Patient Care and Health-Related Costs

Maria Viqar-Syed, MBBS, David J. Bradley, MD, PhD,
Win-Kuang Shen, MD*

KEYWORDS

- Syncope management unit • Emergency department • Health care cost analysis

KEY POINTS

- Clinical studies in several countries have demonstrated that it is possible to design syncope management units (SMUs) with trained personnel to follow clinical pathways based on recommendations from multidisciplinary societies such as the European Society of Cardiology (ESC), the American College of Emergency Physicians (ACEP), the American Heart Association (AHA), the American College of Cardiology (ACC), and the American College of Physicians.
- The ideal SMU should have resources for interdisciplinary testing and consultations available in a timely manner. The specific operational organization of the SMU may vary from hospital to hospital.
- Most studies have reported clinical outcomes from large hospitals or tertiary care centers; future studies must be from SMUs in community hospitals where multidisciplinary teams may not be readily available.
- SMUs decrease the rate of hospitalization for syncope. Future studies will clarify whether SMU-associated reductions in hospitalization translate into SMUs being cost-effective compared with usual care.

INTRODUCTION

Syncope is a self-resolving event characterized by the loss of consciousness due to transient global cerebral hypoperfusion. Quick onset, short duration, and spontaneous complete recovery are hallmarks that sometimes pose a challenge to the management of syncope. The estimated incidence of syncope is 6.2 per 1000 person-years in the Framingham study and is the same among men and women.[1] Syncope is a common presentation in general practice.[2]

Clinical decision making can be challenging in the emergency department (ED)[3] management of patients with recent syncope. Most patients are asymptomatic on arrival in the ED. As a definitive diagnosis often cannot be determined in the time frame available in the ED and because syncope may be a harbinger of sudden death among patients with increased risk of cardiac syncope, physicians often take a "safe" approach when managing high- and intermediate-risk patients by admitting most of these patients to the hospital.[4] Although the rationale of this approach is understandable, the presumption that in-hospital evaluation improves a patient's clinical outcome has never been demonstrated.

The lack of a standard syncope evaluation pathway and the concern of not recognizing a potentially life-threatening cause of syncope frequently lead to multiple diagnostic tests being ordered to

Division of Cardiovascular Diseases, Department of Internal Medicine, Mayo Clinic Arizona, Mayo Clinic College of Medicine, 200 1st Street Southwest, Rochester, MN, USA
* Corresponding author.
E-mail address: wshen@mayo.edu

Cardiol Clin 31 (2013) 39–49
http://dx.doi.org/10.1016/j.ccl.2012.10.006
0733-8651/13/$ – see front matter © 2013 Elsevier Inc. All rights reserved.

rule out different causes of syncope. The combination of high hospital admissions and multiple diagnostic tests contribute to the high cost of syncope care. More than $2 billion a year is spent in acute care facilities in the United States for the evaluation of patients with syncope.[5]

Syncope guidelines from the ESC[6] and clinical policy and position statements from the ACEP,[4] AHA/ACC Foundation,[7] and American College of Physicians[8,9] have made recommendations to risk stratify and systematize management of patients with syncope. Despite these published guidelines and position statements, hospitalization admission rates for patients presenting to EDs with recent syncope remain high, and the use of multiple testing continues to be frequent.[10–12]

The concept of an SMU in the ED (or in other inpatient or outpatient settings) originated from the question of whether a specialized unit designated for syncope evaluation could increase diagnostic outcomes and decrease hospital admission rates. A related question was whether a syncope unit practice model would affect patients' short- and long-term outcomes with regard to recurrent syncope and mortality.[13] If a specialized syncope unit could be effective and efficient in managing patients with syncope, how would such a practice affect the cost of health care of this large patient population? This review provides a summary of how the syncope unit has affected clinical outcomes and health-related costs.

EVIDENCE OF HIGH HOSPITAL ADMISSION RATES FOR SYNCOPE

Syncope not only accounts for 1% of ED presentations[10,14] in adults older than 65 years but also is the sixth most common cause of hospital admissions.[15,16] During syncope evaluation, the first goal is to establish the cause of syncope. Treatment is implemented according to the cause of syncope. The risk of recurrent syncope is related to the cause of syncope and the effectiveness of the therapy. The prognosis of patients after syncope is a function of the type and severity of the underlying disease.

The goals of evaluation of patients in the ED are to stratify patients with respect to risk of cardiac mortality and morbidity and to determine the cause of syncope in a timely manner. The risk of syncope due to cardiac causes could be as high as 21%.[11] ED physicians evaluating patients with syncope often face a challenge in deciding which patients may require immediate hospital admission and which patients can be safely discharged from the ED to be followed up in an outpatient setting.

In a validation study,[17] investigators sought to define the application of ESC guidelines to hospital admissions and discharge in the ED. Of 1124 patients with syncope, 566 were admitted and 558 discharged (50% in each group). Of the 1124 patients, 440 met admission criteria according to the guidelines by ESC, of whom 393(89%) were admitted. Of the 1124 patients, 684 did not meet the criteria for admission, but only 511(75%) were discharged. Appropriateness for admission via the ED according to ESC guidelines was only 69%. These findings suggested that a significantly higher number of hospital admissions occurred in the real world of clinical practice despite many patients not meeting admission criteria. Although ESC guidelines were implemented in these hospitals, there is room for improvement with more rigorous adherence to guidelines. The overuse of hospital admissions could be due to insufficient training or a lack of a care system with expertise in managing patients with syncope.

SYNCOPE MANAGEMENT UNITS

The SMU was developed based on the hypothesis that a specialized syncope unit equipped with diagnostic resources and a multidisciplinary team would improve the diagnostic yield and reduce hospital admission rates compared with standard care (controls) at the conclusion of the ED evaluation. Several models of the SMU are summarized in **Table 1**.

Syncope Unit in the Emergency Department

The Syncope Evaluation in the Emergency Department Study (SEEDS)[13] was a prospective, randomized, single-center study in North America in a tertiary medical center. Patients were risk stratified for cardiovascular morbidity and mortality according to the ACEP clinical policy statement and were divided into high-, intermediate-, and low-risk groups (**Table 2**). Of the 263 patients who consented, 70 high-risk patients were hospitalized for inpatient management and 90 low-risk patients were discharged from the ED. Of 103 intermediate-risk patients, 51 were randomized to evaluation in the ED-based SMU and 52 to standard care.

SMU-randomized patients received continuous cardiac telemetry for up to 6 hours and orthostatic blood pressure (BP) monitoring and were eligible for further testing, if indicated. This additional testing included echocardiography, tilt-table testing, and electrophysiologic consultation. The probable diagnosis was established in 34 (67%) patients randomized to the SMU group and in 5 (10%) patients randomized to the standard care group (*P*<.001); hospital admission was required for 22 (43%) and 51 (98%) patients, respectively (*P*<.001). SEEDS showed that an ED-based SMU equipped with suitable resources and multidisciplinary teamwork improves diagnostic yield and decreases hospitalization without adversely affecting measured clinical outcomes.

Syncope Unit in the Hospital

Brignole and colleagues[10] compared hospitals equipped with a syncope unit with matched hospitals without such facilities and enrolled patients with syncope for management. There were 279 patients in the 6 syncope unit hospitals and 274 in the 6 control hospitals. Hospitals were equipped with tools for diagnosing syncope, such as tilt-table testing, cardiac telemetry, and electrophysiologic and neurologic testing. Only 30 (11%) patients were referred to the syncope unit in the study group for assessment. There was no statistically significant difference between syncope unit patients compared with control patients in hospitalization rate (43% vs 49%, *P* = NS) or tests performed (3.3 ± 2.2 vs 3.6 ± 2.2 per patient, *P* = NS). The syncope unit patients underwent fewer basic laboratory tests (75% vs 86%, *P* = .002), brain-imaging investigations (17% vs 24%, *P* = .05), and echocardiograms (11% vs 16%, *P* = .04) and more carotid sinus massage (13% vs 8%, *P* = .03) and tilt testing (8% vs 1%, *P* = .000). Investigations were performed by keeping the ESC guidelines in view. Syncope units affected overall management, and fewer tests such as echocardiograms and magnetic resonance imaging were performed. Hospitals with SMUs used recommendations by the ESC more effectively in the few patients who were referred to them.

Outpatient Syncope Referral Unit

Another model of care is an outpatient secondary referral center,[18] which consists of a multidisciplinary group including cardiologists and specialist nurses with experience in arrhythmias, falls, and epilepsy. Evidence-based Web algorithms are incorporated in care pathways for the management of patients, with special emphasis on differential diagnosis between syncope, epilepsy, and psychogenic episodes. A specialist nurse-led Rapid Access Blackouts Triage Clinic (RABTC) efficiently risk stratified patients and directed management after making the initial diagnosis. A total of 327 patients were studied. Referral to assessment time was 35 ± 19 (median 31) days. About 60% of patients fell into the high-risk category because of one or more high-risk features: abnormal

electrocardiogram (ECG), personal or family history of sudden cardiac death, syncope during exercise, new neurologic deficit, and history suggestive of epilepsy or brain injury. In patients whose syncope type was uncertain, further appropriate testing was performed and referrals to neurology, electrophysiology for pacing needs, and other disciples were made. The diagnosis and management plans were delivered within the RABTC for 144 patients (44%). Thirty-nine patients (12%) were discharged to primary care with reassurance, and 31 (10%) were referred on for detailed specialist evaluation, mostly neurologic (26/31, 84%). Readmission rates decreased after evaluation in the clinic (from 46.2% to 6.8%, *P*<.001), and there was no difference in the follow-up time, readmission, or discharge rates between high- and low-risk patients.

The Falls and Syncope Service (FASS)[19] is a rapid access, multidisciplinary approach for adult and elderly patients with syncope presenting to the ED in England. FASS has the capability of performing tilt testing, beat-to-beat BP monitoring, and ambulatory monitoring, as well as physiotherapy, occupational therapy, and specialist nursing skills. All patients have an initial detailed assessment by a physician with falls and syncope interest and expertise and are managed by FASS or neurology, cardiology, or otolaryngology department, depending on the findings at the initial assessment. In this study, 388 patients were prospectively studied at baseline for demographics, investigations, diagnoses, readmission rates, length of hospital stay, assessments of gait and balance, and FASS referrals. After 1 year, a second audit of 379 prospective patients was performed after intervention with introduction of Web-based algorithms. These teaching algorithms were visible in clinical areas as well as educational lectures, providing an outline for history taking, examination, and investigations, along with directions for inpatient versus outpatient management and subspecialty referrals.

The total number of admissions with falls and syncope was reduced (10.6% vs 8.2%, *P* = NS). The rate of readmission within 30 days also decreased. Clinical investigations decreased at second audit, with fewer cardiological (*P* = .0003) and neurologic investigations. Gait and balance were recorded more frequently (20% vs 52%, *P* = .006). ECG, echocardiography, and electroencephalography were less frequently requested. Referral to FASS tended to decrease (10% vs 6%, *P* = NS). The general physicians rather than the subspecialists diagnosed neurocardiogenic syncope at the second audit.

Thus, FASS showed that evidence-based algorithms for syncope that advised for admission,

Table 1
Models of syncope management unit

Syncope Unit Setting	Study Design	Patient Demographics	Findings	Comments
Syncope unit in the hospital[10]	Prospective, cohort study, 6 hospitals equipped with a syncope unit and 6 matched hospitals without a syncope unit	279 study patients vs 274 control patients	Less hospitalizations and tests in study patients Carotid sinus massage and tilt testing was performed more frequently In study patients neurally mediated syncope was more commonly diagnosed	Standardized approach for the management of syncope is effective Syncope unit should coordinate management closely with ED
Syncope unit in emergency department[13]	Prospective, randomized, single-center study comparing outcomes with syncope unit management in ED vs standard management.	51 study patients vs 52 control patients	Superior diagnostic yield and decreased hospitalization for study patients (P<.001)	Syncope unit in ED increases diagnostic yield and decreases hospitalizations without affecting all-cause mortality in a cost-efficient manner
Functional syncope unit with general internal medicine services[19]	Observational prospective study with baseline audit and repeat audit after 1 year after intervention with Falls and Syncope Services (FASS) model. Care followed evidence-based algorithms with initial testing at first visit, and appropriate referrals to subspecialists	388 baseline patients and 379 patients at 1 y managed with Web-based algorithms	23% overall reduction in hospital admission with fewer cardiological (P = .0003) and neurologic investigations and more frequent gait and balance recorded (P = .0006) at second audit. 19% fewer patients admitted from home while more nursing home patients admitted at second audit	Following algorithms directed toward guidance for testing, need for admission, and referrals resulted in better use of resources

Syncope unit in the hospital[58]	Retrospective study of patients managed under FASS model of care (The Newcastle Rapid Access FASS in elderly)	180 patients, older than 65 y	High diagnostic yield (92.5%) and reduced hospital days. Vasovagal syncope was a frequent cause in elderly people (37%). Falls were seen in 11%	Syncope services led by geriatricians are beneficial in elderly patients
Syncope unit in the outpatient clinic[18]	Secondary referral center Specialist nurse-led therapy Access Blackouts Triage Clinic, with the use of Web-based algorithms to direct patients in different care pathways	327 study patients	Patients were seen within 35 ± 19 d of referral >50% of patients were diagnosed with structured clinical triage based on Web algorithm and ECG Data discussed with a cardiologist if needed and referral to other specialists and testing as appropriate	RABTC as a bridge between first responders and specialist referral Evaluation through an RABTC; reduced readmissions (46.2% vs 6.8%, $P<.001$)

Table 2
ED risk stratification of patients with syncope in SEEDS

High-Risk Group	Intermediate-Risk Group	Low-Risk Group
Chest pain compatible with acute coronary syndrome	Age ≥50 y	Age <50 y
Signs of congestive heart failure	With previous history of Coronary artery disease Myocardial infarction Congestive heart failure Cardiomyopathy without active symptoms or signs On cardiac medications Bundle-branch block or Q wave without acute changes on ECG	With no previous history of cardiovascular disease
Moderate/severe valvular disease	Family history of premature (<50 y), unexplained sudden death	Symptoms consistent with reflex-mediated or vasovagal syncope
History of ventricular arrhythmias	Symptoms not consistent with a reflex-mediated or vasovagal cause	Normal cardiovascular examination
ECG/cardiac monitor findings of ischemia	Cardiac devices without evidence of dysfunction	Normal ECG findings
Prolonged QTc (≥500 ms)	Physician's judgment that suspicion of cardiac syncope is reasonable	
Trifascicular block or pauses between 2 and 3 s		
Persistent sinus bradycardia between 40 and 60 bpm		
Atrial fibrillation and nonsustained ventricular tachycardia without symptoms		
Cardiac devices (pacemaker or defibrillator) with dysfunction		

Data from Shen WK, Decker WW, Smars PA, et al. Syncope Evaluation in the Emergency Department Study (SEEDS). A multidisciplinary approach to syncope management. Circulation 2004;110(24):3636–45.

investigations, and referrals resulted in correct diagnosis, effective management, and reduced readmission rates due to syncope and implemented good medical practices.

Effective Core Elements of Syncope Management Units

What are the elements in the SMU that are critical for its success? Syncope evaluation begins with risk stratification. The various schemes of stratification are reviewed by Furlan and colleagues elsewhere in this issue, and a proposed syncope management model from the ED to the hospital is shown in **Fig. 1**. Properly trained staff who are familiar with the validated and standardized risk stratification protocols are an important element of a specialized syncope unit to conduct effective,

efficient, and appropriate decisions for hospital admission and subsequent testing. Who should be the trained staff in the SMU? Subspecialty practices are more prevalent in the United States in general and in large tertiary medical centers. In the SEEDS investigation, electrophysiologists and ED specialists in a large tertiary center in the United States led the team. In Italy, experienced cardiologists or physicians with special interests in syncope directed the model. In the FASS model in the United Kingdom, geriatricians and internists with expertise in syncope and falls lead the syncope team. In the RABTC model in the United Kingdom, a well-trained nursing team directs the outpatient clinic. Regardless of who may be the "team leader," it is clear that the team leader must have expertise in syncope evaluation and management and the syncope unit team requires

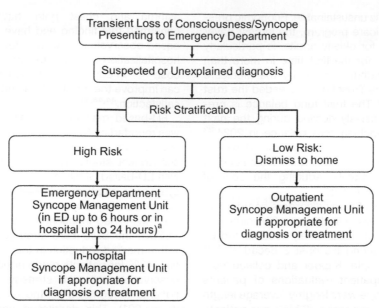

Fig. 1. A proposed syncope management model from the emergency department to the hospital. [a] The 6-hour ED syncope unit evaluation was examined and validated in the SEEDS study. The 24-hour hospital syncope unit evaluation proposed is primarily based on 2 factors. Within 24 hours, the medical team should decide whether the patient needs to remain in the hospital for further evaluation/therapy or is ready for dismissal and outpatient management. When a hospital stay is 24 hours or less, the patient can be managed under the "observational" status without "being admitted," thereby potentially reducing health care resource use. (*Modified from* Brignole M, Shen WK. Syncope management from emergency department to hospital. J Am Coll Cardiol 2008;51(3):284–7; with permission.)

a multidisciplinary approach, as the patient population is diverse. Specialists in cardiology, electrophysiology, neurology, and other disciplines should be available if a consultation is required.

What are the tests essential in the syncope unit? Although diagnostic yield is low, most practices would consider complete blood count and ECG as routine baseline testing. A thorough history and physical examination including carotid sinus massage in elderly patients (without contraindications) and orthostatic BP checks are part of the initial evaluation. Continuous and prolonged rhythm monitoring, echocardiography, tilt-table testing, and treadmill exercise testing should be available at the syncope unit team's discretion. Additional and advanced cardiac or neurologic testing may vary as a function of regional practice.

Ultimately, the "comfort" level of physicians' decision regarding hospital admission versus outpatient evaluation in patients with intermediate risk of prognosis depends on the availability of follow-up arrangements after the initial ED or hospital evaluation. In the SEEDS study, patients dismissed from ED were seen at the outpatient Arrhythmia Clinic within 72 hours if deemed appropriate. This requirement was part of the study

design and likely contributed to the decrease in hospital admission. In the FASS and RABTC studies, outpatient teams with expertise in syncope evaluation were available to guide triaging and subsequent evaluation. Outcomes from these models suggest that a specialized outpatient clinic capable of seeing patients for initial evaluation or for follow-up after dismissal from the ED or hospital in a timely manner is an important component in the syncope unit practice model.

HEALTH CARE ECONOMICS

The financial and quality challenges facing the US health care system are well documented. US health care expenditures as a share of the gross domestic product (GDP) increased from 7.4% in 1972 to 17.6% in 2010, making the United States by far the leader among all countries in health care outlays as a proportion of GDP.[20] Despite this huge investment in health care, the United States ranks only 25th among industrialized countries in one key statistic: life expectancy.[21] The ability of the United States to pay ever-greater amounts for advancing health technology for an aging population is unsustainable. Economic pressure on the Medicare program, the largest payer for medical care for elderly adults, is particularly intense. In 2011, for the first time in more than a decade, expenditures made by the Medicare Hospital Insurance Trust Fund exceeded the trust fund's income.[22] The trust fund balance is predicted to progressively decline during the next several years, reaching zero balance in 2024.[22] More pessimistic assessments predict depletion of the Medicare Hospital Insurance Trust Fund as early as 2017.[22] Safely reducing the cost of medical care is imperative.

Syncope is one of many disorders contributing to the financial crisis in health care. The high cost of syncope evaluation has been documented by several studies during the past 3 decades.[23–37] In 1982, for example, Kapoor and colleagues[33] reported that inpatient evaluations of patients with recent syncope were lengthy (average length of stay, 9 days), expensive ($2463 per patient), and of low yield (cause of syncope diagnosed in 13 of 121 patients). Calkins and colleagues,[26] in 1993, showed that, even for patients with a history strongly suggestive of vasovagal syncope, the cost of syncope evaluation was high ($3763 per patient). Because the cause of a given episode of syncope may initially be unclear and because syncope can on occasion be caused by a life-threatening problem such as ventricular arrhythmias, physicians may have a tendency to err on the side of caution by hospitalizing a large proportion of patients with syncope. Between 2000 and 2010, the number of patients hospitalized with a diagnosis of syncope in the United States (ICD-9780.2) increased by 30% from to 462,000 to 602,000. Sun and colleagues[5] showed in 2005 that the yearly cost of syncope-related inpatient care in the United States was 2.4 billion dollars. Enhancing the ability of physicians to identify patients who can safely undergo evaluation of syncope on a less costly outpatient basis may substantially reduce the cost of syncope care.

Assessment of patients with recent syncope in a specialized evaluation unit, such as an ED-based SMU, holds promise of reducing hospital admissions and costs and possibly improving outcomes for patients with syncope. ED-based management units or observation units provide additional monitoring and testing for selected patients.[38,39] In 1976, Diamond and colleagues[40] reported their experience with an ED-based observation unit in Los Angeles. They noted that "the cost for patient care [in an observation ward] is considerably lower than [the cost for] inpatient service." Several studies, focusing mainly on asthma and chest pain, have subsequently confirmed this finding and have shown that ED-based observation units can decrease the rate of hospitalization, length of inpatient stay, and cost.[40–47] In addition, ED-based observation units can improve the quality of life and increase patient satisfaction.[44,46,48]

ED-based management unit care for syncope was reported by Brillman and colleagues[49] in 1995 and by Cunningham and Mikhail[50] in 2001. Several subsequent studies have described experiences with ED-based SMUs as well as other specialized syncope evaluation units.[10,13,15,17,25,51–56] Use of a specialized syncope evaluation unit is associated with decreased inpatient length of stay.[13,15,54] In SEEDS, the SMU care strategy was associated with a marked reduction in the rate of hospitalization: 43% for patients randomized to the syncope observation unit care strategy versus 98% for patients randomized to the usual care strategy ($P = .001$). This decreased hospitalization rate was associated with a decrease in total patient-hospital days from 140 to 64. Although there was no statistically significant difference in survival between patients in the 2 arms of the trial (**Fig. 2**), the study was not designed and powered to compare survival. Among patients randomized to the SMU care strategy, there was a greater use of outpatient resources for the index syncopal episode as well as increased use of tilt-table testing. Quality of life and utilities were not measured.

Can one conclude that ED-based SMUs are cost-effective compared with usual care among patients with intermediate syncope risk presenting to US EDs? This question would ideally be answered by an adequately powered randomized trial in which costs, survival, and utilities were measured prospectively among patients randomized to syncope unit care versus usual care.[57] With such data in hand, an assessment of the incremental cost-effectiveness ratio of the syncope unit strategy versus the standard care strategy could be estimated in dollars per quality adjusted life year gained. If this incremental cost-effectiveness ratio and its associated degree of uncertainty were economically attractive (eg, less than $100,000 for every quality adjusted life year gained), one could conclude that ED-based SMUs are cost-effective compared with usual care. Although specialized syncope unit evaluation plausibly decreases the use of inpatient resources, inpatient savings may be partially or entirely offset by SMU costs and outpatient costs. Additional data and analyses are needed before conclusions can be drawn about whether SMUs are cost-effective compared with usual care in dollars per quality adjusted life year gained.

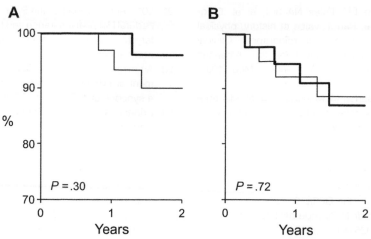

Fig. 2. Long-term clinical outcomes from SEEDS. (*A*) Survival free from death; (*B*) survival free from recurrent syncope. Bold line represents syncope unit group; standard line represents standard care group. The probability of survival at 2 years was 97% for the syncope unit group and 90% for the standard care group (P0.30). Recurrent syncope was reported in 9 patients (4 in the syncope unit group). The probability of being free of a syncopal event at 2 years was 88% for the syncope unit group and 89% for the standard care group (P0.72). (*Modified from* Shen WK, Decker WW, Smars PA, et al. Syncope Evaluation in the Emergency Department Study (SEEDS). A multidisciplinary approach to syncope management. Circulation 2004;110(24):3636–45; with permission.)

SUMMARY

Outcomes from clinical studies from several countries have demonstrated that it is possible to design syncope units with trained personnel to follow clinical pathways based on recommendations from multidisciplinary societies such as the ESC, ACEP, AHA, ACC, and American College of Physicians. The ideal SMU should have resources for interdisciplinary testing and consultations available in a timely manner. The specific operational organization of the SMU may vary from hospital to hospital or region to region according to local practice models, available personnel, and/or health care resources. Most studies have reported clinical outcomes from large hospitals or tertiary care centers. Future studies must be from SMUs in community hospitals where multidisciplinary teams may not be readily available. SMUs decrease the rate of hospitalization for syncope. Future studies are needed to clarify whether SMU-associated reductions in hospitalization translate into SMUs being cost-effective compared with usual care.

REFERENCES

1. Soteriades ES, Evans JC, Larson MG, et al. Incidence and prognosis of syncope. N Engl J Med 2002;347(12):878–85.
2. Olde Nordkamp LR, van Dijk N, Ganzeboom KS, et al. Syncope prevalence in the ED compared to general practice and population: a strong selection process. Am J Emerg Med 2009;27(3):271–9.
3. Moya A, Sutton R, Ammirati F, et al. Guidelines for the diagnosis and management of syncope (version 2009). Eur Heart J 2009;30(21):2631–71.
4. Huff JS, Decker WW, Quinn JV, et al. Clinical policy: critical issues in the evaluation and management of adult patients presenting to the emergency department with syncope. Ann Emerg Med 2007;49(4):431–44.
5. Sun BC, Emond JA, Camargo CA Jr. Direct medical costs of syncope-related hospitalizations in the United States. Am J Cardiol 2005;95(5):668–71.
6. The European Society of Cardiology guidelines for the diagnosis and management of syncope reviewed by Angel Moya, MD, FESC, Chair of the Guideline Task Force with J. Taylor, MPhil. Eur Heart J 2009;30(21):2539–40.
7. Strickberger SA, Benson DW, Biaggioni I, et al. AHA/ACCF Scientific Statement on the evaluation of syncope: from the American Heart Association Councils on Clinical Cardiology, Cardiovascular Nursing, Cardiovascular Disease in the Young, and Stroke, and the Quality of Care and Outcomes Research Interdisciplinary Working Group; and the American College of Cardiology Foundation: in collaboration with the Heart Rhythm Society: endorsed by the American Autonomic Society. Circulation 2006;113(2):316–27.
8. Linzer M, Yang EH, Estes NA 3rd, et al. Diagnosing syncope. Part 2: unexplained syncope. Clinical efficacy assessment project of the American College of Physicians. Ann Intern Med 1997;127(1):76–86.

9. Linzer M, Yang EH, Estes NA 3rd, et al. Diagnosing syncope. Part 1: value of history, physical examination, and electrocardiography. Clinical efficacy assessment project of the American College of Physicians. Ann Intern Med 1997; 126(12):989–96.

10. Brignole M, Disertori M, Menozzi C, et al. Management of syncope referred urgently to general hospitals with and without syncope units. Europace 2003; 5(3):293–8.

11. Ammirati F, Colivicchi F, Santini M. Diagnosing syncope in clinical practice. Implementation of a simplified diagnostic algorithm in a multicentre prospective trial - the OESIL 2 study (Osservatorio Epidemiologico della Sincope nel Lazio). Eur Heart J 2000;21(11):935–40.

12. Elesber AA, Decker WW, Smars PA, et al. Impact of the application of the American College of Emergency Physicians recommendations for the admission of patients with syncope on a retrospectively studied population presenting to the emergency department. Am Heart J 2005;149(5):826–31.

13. Shen WK, Decker WW, Smars PA, et al. Syncope evaluation in the emergency department study (SEEDS). A multidisciplinary approach to syncope management. Circulation 2004;110(24):3636–45.

14. Blanc JJ, L'Her C, Touiza A, et al. Prospective evaluation and outcome of patients admitted for syncope over a 1 year period. Eur Heart J 2002; 23(10):815–20.

15. Kenny RA, O'Shea D, Walker HF. Impact of a dedicated syncope and falls facility for older adults on emergency beds. Age Ageing 2002;31(4):272–5.

16. Thijs RD, Wieling W, Kaufmann H, et al. Defining and classifying syncope. Clin Auton Res 2004; 14(Suppl 1):4–8.

17. Bartoletti A, Fabiani P, Adriani P, et al. Hospital admission of patients referred to the emergency department for syncope: a single-hospital prospective study based on the application of the European Society of Cardiology guidelines on syncope. Eur Heart J 2006;27(1):83–8.

18. Petkar S, Bell W, Rice N, et al. Initial experience with a rapid access blackouts triage clinic. Clin Med 2011;11(1):11–6.

19. Parry SW, Frearson R, Steen N, et al. Evidence-based algorithms and the management of falls and syncope presenting to acute medical services. Clin Med 2008;8(2):157–62.

20. Organisation for Economic Co-operation and Development. Available at: http://www.oecd-ilibrary.org/social-issues-migration-health/total-expenditure-on-health_20758480-table1. Accessed August 25, 2012.

21. OECD. Life expectancy at birth, total population, Health: Key Tables from OECD, No. 8. 2012. http://dx.doi.org/10.1787/lifexpy-total-table-2012-1-en. Accessed August 25, 2012.

22. 2012 Annual report of the Boards of Trustees of the Federal Hospital Insurance and Federal Supplementary Medical Insurance Trust Funds. Annual report proceedings 2012.

23. Ammirati F, Colaceci R, Cesario A, et al. Management of syncope: clinical and economic impact of a syncope unit. Europace 2008;10(4):471–6.

24. Brignole M, Ungar A, Bartoletti A, et al. Standardized-care pathway vs. usual management of syncope patients presenting as emergencies at general hospitals. Europace 2006;8(8):644–50.

25. Brignole M, Ungar A, Casagranda I, et al. Prospective multicentre systematic guideline-based management of patients referred to the syncope units of general hospitals. Europace 2010;12(1):109–18.

26. Calkins H, Byrne M, el-Atassi R, et al. The economic burden of unrecognized vasodepressor syncope. Am J Med 1993;95(5):473–9.

27. Casini-Raggi V, Bandinelli G, Lagi A. Vasovagal syncope in emergency room patients: analysis of a metropolitan area registry. Neuroepidemiology 2002;21:287–91.

28. Del Greco M, Cozzio S, Scillieri M, et al. Diagnostic pathway of syncope and analysis of the impact of guidelines in a district general hospital. The ECSIT study (Epidemiology and Costs of Syncope in Trento). Ital Heart J 2003;4(2):99–106.

29. Eagle KA, Black HR. The impact of diagnostic tests in evaluating patients with syncope. Yale J Biol Med 1983;56(1):1–8.

30. Farwell D, Sulke N. How do we diagnose syncope? J Cardiovasc Electrophysiol 2002;13:S9–13.

31. Farwell DJ, Freemantle N, Sulke AN. Use of implantable loop recorders in the diagnosis and management of syncope. Eur Heart J 2004;25(14):1257–63.

32. Gordon TA, Moodie DS, Passalacqua M, et al. A retrospective analysis of the cost-effective workup of syncope in children. Cleve Clin J Med 1987;54(5): 391–4.

33. Kapoor WN, Karpf M, Maher Y, et al. Syncope of unknown origin. The need for a more cost-effective approach to its diagnosis evaluation. JAMA 1982; 247(19):2687–91.

34. Krahn AD, Klein GJ, Yee R, et al. Cost implications of testing strategy in patients with syncope: randomized assessment of syncope trial. J Am Coll Cardiol 2003;42(3):495–501.

35. Mendu ML, McAvay G, Lampert R, et al. Yield of diagnostic tests in evaluating syncopal episodes in older patients. Arch Intern Med 2009;169(14):1299–305.

36. Nyman JA, Krahn AD, Bland PC, et al. The costs of recurrent syncope of unknown origin in elderly patients. Pacing Clin Electrophysiol 1999;22(9): 1386–94.

37. Schillinger M, Domanovits H, Mullner M, et al. Admission for syncope: evaluation, cost and prognosis. Wien Klin Wochenschr 2000;112(19):835–41.

38. Bobzien WF 3rd. The observation-holding area; a prospective study. JACEP 1979;8(12):508–12.
39. Hostetler B, Leikin JB, Timmons JA, et al. Patterns of use of an emergency department-based observation unit. Am J Ther 2002;9(6):499–502.
40. Diamond NJ, Schofferman JA, Elliot JW. Evaluation of an emergency department observation ward. JACEP 1976;5(1):29–31.
41. Farkouh ME, Smars PA, Reeder GS, et al. A clinical trial of a chest-pain observation unit for patients with unstable angina. N Engl J Med 1998;339(26):1882–8.
42. Farrell RG. Use of an observation ward in a community hospital. Ann Emerg Med 1982; 11(7):353–7.
43. Gomez MA, Anderson JL, Karagounis LA, et al. An emergency department-based protocol for rapidly ruling out myocardial ischemia reduces hospital time and expense: results of a randomized study (ROMIO). J Am Coll Cardiol 1996; 28(1):25–33.
44. McDermott MF, Murphy DG, Zalenski RJ, et al. A comparison between emergency diagnostic and treatment unit and inpatient care in the management of acute asthma. Arch Intern Med 1997;157(18): 2055–62.
45. Roberts RR, Zalenski RJ, Mensah EK, et al. Costs of an emergency department-based accelerated diagnostic protocol vs hospitalization in patients with chest pain: a randomized controlled trial. JAMA 1997;278(20):1670–6.
46. Rydman RJ, Isola ML, Roberts RR, et al. Emergency department observation unit versus hospital inpatient care for a chronic asthmatic population: a randomized trial of health status outcome and cost. Med Care 1998;36(4):599–609.
47. Zwicke DL, Donohue JF, Wagner EH. Use of the emergency department observation unit in the treatment of acute asthma. Ann Emerg Med 1982;11(2): 77–83.
48. Rydman RJ, Roberts RR, Albrecht GL, et al. Patient satisfaction with an emergency department asthma observation unit. Acad Emerg Med 1999; 6(3):178–83.
49. Brillman J, Mathers-Dunbar L, Graff L, et al. Management of observation units. American College of Emergency Physicians. Ann Emerg Med 1995; 25(6):823–30.
50. Cunningham R, Mikhail MG. Management of patients with syncope and cardiac arrhythmias in an emergency department observation unit. Emerg Med Clin North Am 2001;19(1):105–21, vii.
51. Bartoletti A, Fabiani P, Bagnoli L, et al. Physical injuries caused by a transient loss of consciousness: main clinical characteristics of patients and diagnostic contribution of carotid sinus massage. Eur Heart J 2008;29(5):618–24.
52. Iglesias JF, Graf D, Forclaz A, et al. Stepwise evaluation of unexplained syncope in a large ambulatory population. Pacing Clin Electrophysiol 2009; 32(Suppl 1):S202–6.
53. McCarthy F, McMahon CG, Geary U, et al. Management of syncope in the emergency department: a single hospital observational case series based on the application of European Society of Cardiology guidelines. Europace 2009;11(2):216–24.
54. Numeroso F, Mossini G, Spaggiari E, et al. Syncope in the emergency department of a large northern Italian hospital: incidence, efficacy of a short-stay observation ward and validation of the OESIL risk score. Emerg Med J 2010;27(9):653–8.
55. Petkar S, Bell W, Rice N, et al. Rationale for a rapid access blackouts triage clinic. Br J Card Nurs 2008; 10:468–74.
56. Ross MA, Compton S, Richardson D, et al. The use and effectiveness of an emergency department observation unit for elderly patients. Ann Emerg Med 2003;41(5):668–77.
57. Gold MR, Siegel JE, Russell LB, et al, editors. Cost-effectiveness in health and medicine. USA: Oxford University Press; 1996.
58. Newton JL, Marsh A, Frith J, et al. Experience of a rapid access blackout service for older people. Age Ageing 2010;39(2):265–8.

Recognizing Life-Threatening Causes of Syncope

Clarence Khoo, MD[a], Santabhanu Chakrabarti, MD[a],
Laura Arbour, MD[b], Andrew D. Krahn, MD[a],*

KEYWORDS

- Syncope • Clinical history • Cardiac arrest • Structural heart disease • Risk • Repolarization
- Family history • Ventricular arrhythmia

KEY POINTS

- The identification of potentially fatal causes of syncope is usually possible with a careful history and an electrocardiogram (ECG).
- The history should focus on the presence of structural heart disease, leading to the assumption that life-threatening ventricular arrhythmias may have caused syncope if present.
- Uncommon but concerning causes of syncope, including genetic causes, will often be evident based on an unusual context of syncope, a family history of suspicious events, and a careful evaluation of the ECG.
- Tailored investigations stemming from the initial clinical evaluation will confirm a suspected diagnosis and will rarely uncover an unexpected diagnosis.
- Involvement of specialist cardiology and cardiac electrophysiology services in such cases will help facilitate the selection of appropriate tests and subsequent therapeutic options.

INTRODUCTION

The diagnostic challenges posed by an episode of syncope are manifold. The identification of the cause is often far from straightforward, with a key concern for the small chance that the episode represents a potentially fatal process. Cardiovascular causes of syncope can be classified as either neurally mediated or attributable to cardiac abnormality. Cardiac causes of syncope include arrhythmic disturbances and obstructive cardiac lesions.[1] This distinction between potential attributable causes is of paramount importance because cardiac causes of syncope are associated with adverse outcomes, including an increased risk of death.[2,3] Approximately 35% of the population will experience syncope at some point in their lifetime.[4] As a significant proportion result from neurocardiogenic causes (21%–50%), identifying the small proportion with life-threatening causes is crucial in balancing reasonable reassurance in the vast majority of cases with thoughtful investigation in the remainder.[3,5] Accordingly, this article focuses on life-threatening causes of syncope and a diagnostic approach to facilitate their identification.

PROGNOSIS OF A PATIENT WITH SYNCOPE

Although the overall prognosis of an individual presenting with syncope is favorable, certain features reliably portend a poor prognosis. Chief among these is the identification of either a structural or electrical cardiac etiology for the syncopal episode. In early retrospective analyses of patients with syncope, cardiac syncope was associated with a 21% to 30% mortality rate at 1 year versus 4% to 12% in those with noncardiac syncope.[2,6] A more recent study has suggested a more conservative 15% mortality rate at 1 year in patients with cardiac syncope.[7] In the largest such study to

[a] Division of Cardiology, University of British Columbia, Gordon & Leslie Diamond Health Care Centre, 2775 Laurel Street, Vancouver, British Columbia V5Z 1M9, Canada; [b] Island Medical Program, Department of Medical Genetics, University of British Columbia, 1 Hospital Way, Victoria, British Columbia V8Z 6R5, Canada
* Corresponding author.
E-mail address: akrahn@mail.ubc.ca

Cardiol Clin 31 (2013) 51–66
http://dx.doi.org/10.1016/j.ccl.2012.10.005
0733-8651/13/$ – see front matter © 2013 Elsevier Inc. All rights reserved.

date, cardiac syncope was associated with a 2-fold increase in the risk of death compared with those without a history of syncope, with an approximately 50% 5-year survival.[3] By comparison, patients with neurocardiogenic causes of syncope have a favorable prognosis that is comparable to asymptomatic controls.[3,8] However, this is confounded by the poor correlation of the cause of syncope with the cause of subsequent death. The SCD-HeFT trial identified syncope as a high-risk marker for subsequent mortality, but an implantable cardioverter-defibrillator (ICD) or the use of antiarrhythmic agents did not alter the outcome in a comparison with patients treated with placebo.[9]

Even in the absence of a firm diagnosis of cardiac syncope, the presence of structural cardiac abnormalities or evidence of a primary electrical disorder is associated with a poor prognosis and a hazard ratio (HR) for death of 5.57.[10] On the other hand, a structurally normal heart with a normal electrocardiogram (ECG) is usually associated with a benign etiology for syncope and a favorable prognosis.[10,11] Fundamental to the ability to identify high-risk cases of syncope, therefore, is the ability to effectively recognize, or at the very least infer, the presence of either structural or electrical cardiac anomalies. As these anomalies may be subtle, it is prudent to initially familiarize oneself with potentially lethal causes of syncope.

HIGH-RISK CAUSES OF SYNCOPE AND WHEN TO WORRY

Most cases for which syncope is life threatening are neither difficult to diagnose nor, for that matter, difficult to treat. Such cases represent clear evidence of manifest conduction system disease or ventricular arrhythmias, or a propensity to the same with left ventricular (LV) dysfunction or resting conduction disturbances. This article intentionally minimizes the discussion of these scenarios, because they represent established and familiar management scenarios to the reader, summarized in **Box 1** and **Fig. 1**. Acute ischemic syndromes may produce syncope through multiple mechanisms, and should be ruled out in the appropriate clinical setting. Having said this, they are a distinctly unusual cause of unexplained syncope and seldom warrant more than standard noninvasive clinical exclusion.

Arrhythmic Etiology

Arrhythmias are the most common cause of cardiac syncope, and can be further subdivided into (1) bradyarrhythmias and (2) tachyarrhythmias.[12]

Box 1
Life-threatening causes of syncope that typically present in the context of manifest cardiac disease

- Sinus node dysfunction
  - Syncope is a common presentation, but there is little concern regarding sudden death, typically not life threatening
- Atrioventricular node dysfunction
  - Infranodal atrioventricular block (Mobitz II second-degree block)
  - Complete heart block
  - Alternating bundle branch block
- Ventricular tachyarrhythmias
  - Polymorphic ventricular tachycardia secondary to ischemia
  - Scar-related monomorphic ventricular tachycardia
  - Ventricular fibrillation
- Reduction in stroke volume
  - Mechanical complication
    - Cardiac perforation ± pericardial tamponade
    - Ventricular septal rupture
    - Papillary muscle rupture

Bradyarrhythmias

Bradyarrhythmias can result from dysfunction of the conduction system at any level (see **Box 1**). Atrioventricular (AV) block can occur at the level of the AV node (ie, nodal) or below the AV node (ie, infranodal). This distinction is of importance, as infranodal block is more likely to be associated with the lack of an adequate escape rhythm and a small risk of sudden death.[13] Infranodal AV block is generally typified by the presence of Mobitz II second-degree AV block, or the presence of an escape rhythm with an intraventricular conduction delay or overt bundle branch block. Nodal AV block, on the other hand, is associated with Mobitz I (Wenckebach) second-degree AV block, or the presence of a narrow complex escape rhythm. The presence of alternating bundle branch block morphologies signals an individual at high risk of proceeding to complete heart block. Caution must be observed with apparent Wenckebach AV block in the presence of a wide QRS complex, as the level of block may in fact be infranodal (**Fig. 2**).

Tachyarrhythmias

Both supraventricular and ventricular tachyarrhythmias may result in syncope, with failed vascular

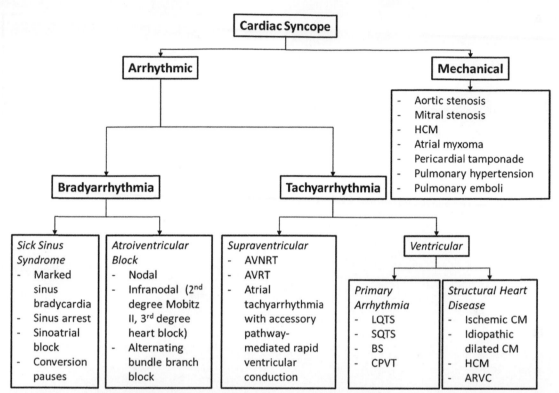

Fig. 1. Flow diagram depicting potential cardiac causes of syncope. AVNRT, atrioventricular nodal reentrant tachycardia; AVRT, atrioventricular reentrant tachycardia; ARVC, arrhythmogenic right ventricular cardiomyopathy; BS, Brugada syndrome; CM, cardiomyopathy; CPVT, catecholaminergic polymorphic ventricular tachycardia; HCM, hypertrophic cardiomyopathy; LQTS, long QT syndrome; SQTS, short QT syndrome.

compensation for the rapid heart rate leading to cerebral hypoperfusion.[1] Ventricular tachyarrhythmias, however, may be sufficiently sustained or may degrade to ventricular fibrillation (VF), resulting in hemodynamic collapse and cardiac arrest. As a result, identification of individuals at risk for ventricular tachyarrhythmias is of paramount importance. This risk is driven by the severity of LV dysfunction, so careful evaluation of LV function is important. Screening history, physical examination, and an ECG are standard, and a transthoracic echocardiogram is warranted if there is any suspicion of heart disease, even though it is seldom diagnostic with respect to syncope.

Individuals with a history of prior myocardial infarction or ventricular dysfunction who present with a syncope history compatible with a cardiac etiology should be evaluated with a high index of suspicion. Even though a left ventricular ejection fraction (LVEF) of less than 40% is associated with a higher risk,[14] the majority of cases of sudden cardiac death (SCD) occur in those with relatively preserved LVEF.[15] As a result, a preserved LVEF should not be used as the sole means of excluding cardiac syncope in a patient with an otherwise suggestive clinical picture.

Where the diagnosis remains unclear, more specialized testing, including surface-averaged ECG, T-wave alternans, exercise testing, cardiac magnetic resonance imaging (MRI) or computed tomography, pharmacologic challenge, or an invasive electrophysiology study may be used for further evaluation (see later discussion).

Primary arrhythmias
Primary life-threatening arrhythmias are uncommon causes of syncope, but represent the worrisome causes that must be detected to prevent tragic sudden death. A comprehensive approach to patient assessment including unique historical clues follows (drowning, exertional or auditory stimuli, and so forth), including "tips and tricks" in detecting these conditions.

Long and short QT syndrome
Long QT syndrome (LQTS) is an inherited ion channelopathy characterized by familial syncope and SCD, which is associated with variable mechanisms of prolonged repolarization measured as QTc prolongation on the ECG. Although more than 12 genes are known to be responsible,[16] the genetic basis is established in the majority of cases

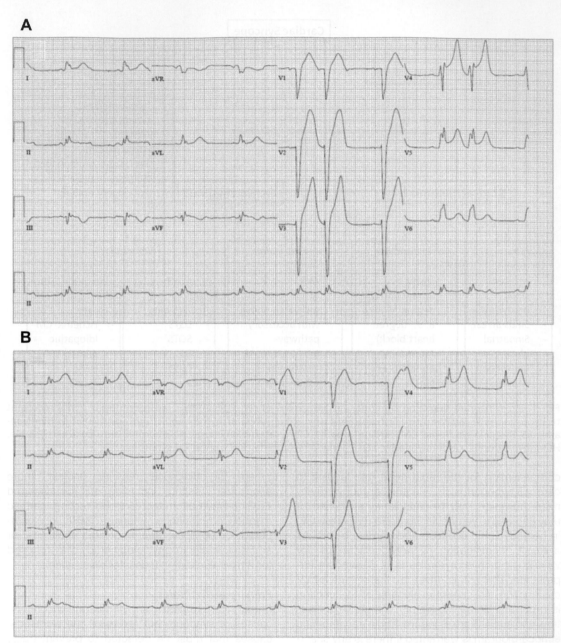

Fig. 2. A patient presenting with bradycardia in the setting of an acute myocardial infarction. (*A*) Mobitz II second-degree heart block with periodic 2:1 atrioventricular conduction. The presence of left bundle branch block and Mobitz II heart block is suggestive of infranodal conduction system disease and a high risk of progression to complete heart block. (*B*) The patient promptly progresses to complete heart block during the same admission.

with mutations in genes encoding potassium-channel proteins (*KCNQ1, KCNH2*). Syncope typically results from a form of polymorphic ventricular tachycardia (VT) classically described as torsades de pointes. The overall prevalence of this group of disorders is 1 in 2500.[17] Common to this group is the presence of a prolonged QTc and abnormal T-wave morphology. Nonetheless, one-third of

cases have a normal or borderline QT interval, and clinical suspicion should drive the pursuit of exercise testing to unmask QT prolongation.[18,19] A QTc greater than 450 milliseconds or >470 milliseconds is considered abnormal in adult males and females, respectively (**Fig. 3**).[20] Historical and ECG features that increase suspicion for LQTS have been identified (**Box 2**).[21,22] In particular, the

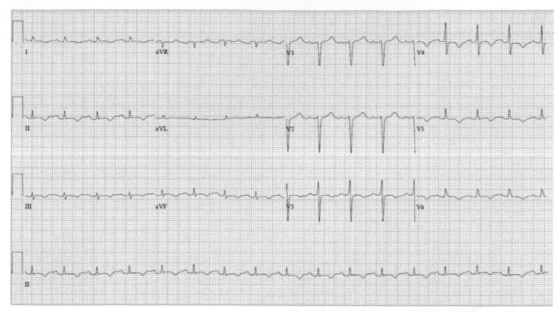

Fig. 3. Twelve-lead electrocardiogram (ECG) of a patient with long QT syndrome diagnosed after sustaining a cardiac arrest. QTc at baseline measured 500 milliseconds. Note that the QT interval is long, and the T-wave morphology is also abnormal.

combination of syncope while supine and a positive family history of SCD provided a positive likelihood ratio of 41 for the diagnosis of LQTS.[22]

Short QT syndrome (SQTS) is the antithesis of LQTS, with overly rapid repolarization leading to QTc less than 300 to 320 milliseconds.[23,24] As with LQTS, SQTS may also present with syncope

and SCD. A gradient of risk for SCD exists, with shorter QTc values associated with a higher risk.[25] Diagnostic criteria for SQTS have been developed incorporating quantitative measures of QTc shortening; clinical factors including history of SCD, VT/VF, unexplained syncope, or atrial fibrillation; a family history of SQTS, SCD, or sudden infant death syndrome; and the presence of a high-risk genotype.[26]

Brugada syndrome

Brugada syndrome (BS) is characterized by anterior precordial ST-segment changes in the context of syncope, cardiac arrest, or sudden death.[27] The prevalence of the ECG pattern ranges from 5 in 10,000 individuals to as high as 12 in 10,000 individuals in Japan.[28,29] Males are predominantly affected, with episodes typically occurring at rest or during sleep, and may be subtly manifest as nocturnal agonal respirations.[30] The ECG of patients with BS is typified by the presence of a right bundle branch block–type conduction pattern with ST elevation in the right precordial leads (**Fig. 4**). Three ECG variants are recognized, but only the type I pattern, which involves at least 2 mm of ST elevation in at least 2 leads of V1 to V3 and an inverted T wave, is diagnostic of BS in the presence of a clinical marker (**Box 3**).[30] It is not uncommon for the ECG to transition from one type to another in the same individual, with triggers including febrile episodes, electrolyte abnormalities, hypothermia, alcohol, or certain drugs.[28] Syncope in this context

---

Box 2
Diagnostic clues for long QT syndrome

History

- Syncope with exertion/emotional stress/supine

- Syncope while sleeping

- Recurrent history of seizures

- Personal or family history of congenital deafness

- Family history of long QT syndrome

- Family history of SCD at age younger than 30 years

ECG

- QTc greater than 450 milliseconds (males), greater than 470 milliseconds (females)

- Documented torsades de pointes

- T-wave alternans

- Notched T waves

- Low heart rate for age

A

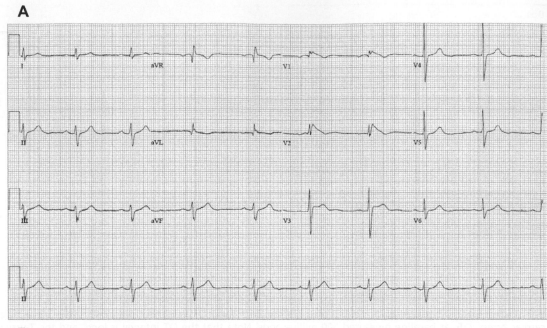

B

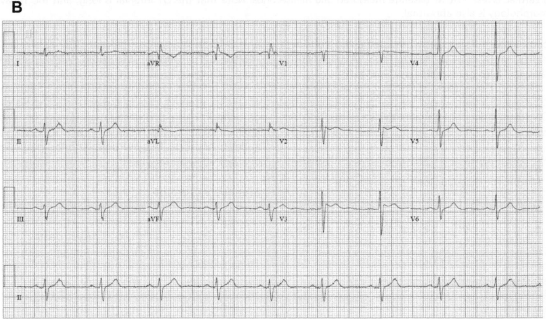

Fig. 4. Series of 12-lead ECGs from a patient with established Brugada syndrome. (*A*) Type I Brugada pattern with ST elevation and inverted T waves in right precordial leads. (*B*) Type II pattern with upright T waves in right precordial leads. This recording was obtained in the same patient on a different day, demonstrating inherent variability of the Brugada ECG pattern.

should raise suspicion of BS. This latter class of triggers includes Class IA antiarrhythmic agents such as procainamide, which may be used as a provocative test to uncover a type I ECG pattern. Use of these drugs (summarized at www.brugadadrugs. org) should be avoided by patients with BS. The simple act of moving the V1 to V3 leads up 1 or 2

intercostal spaces may improve the diagnostic yield of the ECG by unmasking a type I ECG pattern.[31]

Catecholaminergic polymorphic ventricular tachycardia

Catecholaminergic polymorphic VT (CPVT) is characterized by syncope or SCD during exertion

---

Box 3
Diagnostic clues for Brugada syndrome

ECG

- Type I Brugada pattern

  o 2 mm or more ST elevation in at least 2 leads of V1 to V3 and inverted T wave

Clinical

- Documented VT or VF
- Family history of premature SCD
- Family members with type I Brugada pattern
- Inducible VT during electrophysiology study
- Documented syncope
- Nocturnal agonal respirations

---

or with emotional stress, classically caused by the development of bidirectional VT.[32] The majority of individuals have their first presentation before the age of 40 years, though an adult onset associated with a lower incidence of an RyR2 mutation has been described.[33,34] The baseline ECG is usually normal, and the induction of VT by exercise stress testing or epinephrine infusion is the cornerstone in the diagnosis of CPVT. Exercise testing is approximately 80% sensitive in the diagnosis of CPVT.[32]

Wolff-Parkinson-White syndrome and preexcitation

In the presence of symptomatic tachyarrhythmias, individuals with preexcitation may be diagnosed as having the Wolff-Parkinson-White (WPW) syndrome. The risk of SCD with WPW is due to the risk of developing an atrial tachyarrhythmia with rapid conduction to the ventricles over an antegrade-conducting accessory pathway (**Fig. 5**).[35] The mere presence of preexcitation does not immediately indicate a life-threatening cause of syncope, but does identify those who may benefit from further risk stratification in discussion with an electrophysiologist.

Sudden cardiac arrest associated with early repolarization

Although traditionally thought to be a benign variant, early repolarization, defined as 1 mm or more of J-point elevation in at least 2 consecutive inferior or lateral leads (**Fig. 6**), has been shown to be associated with an increased risk for VF.[36–38] However, the link to syncope is tenuous. Given that the early repolarization pattern is not uncommon in the general population, its predictive value for SCD is very low.[37] Until further information

is forthcoming, the presence of early repolarization in a syncopal individual should not be considered contributory.[39]

Inherited and atypical structural heart disease

Hypertrophic cardiomyopathy Hypertrophic cardiomyopathy (HCM) is an autosomal dominant disorder that results in left ventricular hypertrophy (LVH).[40,41] Asymmetric septal hypertrophy leading to dynamic obstruction of the left ventricular outflow tract (LVOT) with exertion is the traditionally described variant, although other patterns may be seen.[42] Even in the absence of outflow tract obstruction, the underlying myocyte disarray and accompanying scarring can serve as the substrate for ventricular tachyarrhythmias. Syncope and SCD may thus result from either arrhythmias or outflow obstruction.[42] The ECG may meet electrocardiographic criteria for LVH, or there may be deep T-wave inversion in the anterior precordial leads, especially in those with apical-dominant involvement. Syncope in a patient with known or suspected HCM should be considered life threatening, and lead to urgent assessment in hospital.

Arrhythmogenic right ventricular cardiomyopathy

Arrhythmogenic right ventricular cardiomyopathy (ARVC) is an autosomal dominant condition with incomplete penetrance that involves fibrofatty replacement of the myocardium, leading to both mechanical ventricular dysfunction and an arrhythmogenic substrate.[43,44] Because mechanical right ventricular disease is typically asymptomatic, ventricular tachyarrhythmias are often the only clinical evidence of disease, leading to palpitations, syncope, or cardiac arrest, even in the presence of only limited structural involvement.[45]

Because of the protean possible manifestations of ARVC and the inherent limitations of diagnostic tests, the diagnosis of ARVC depends on the fulfillment of a combination of major and minor criteria as codified by the 2010 Task Force criteria (**Box 4**).[46–48] Epsilon waves are the classic ECG finding, although T-wave inversion through V1 to V3 has been shown to be a superior diagnostic finding (**Figs. 7** and **8**).[48] Abnormalities of delayed depolarization can be identified by signal-averaged ECG (SAECG)[49,50]; however, the importance of these findings has diminished in the most recent Task Force criteria.[46]

Mechanical Etiology

Obstruction to LV outflow can limit the ability of the heart to increase its cardiac output to meet

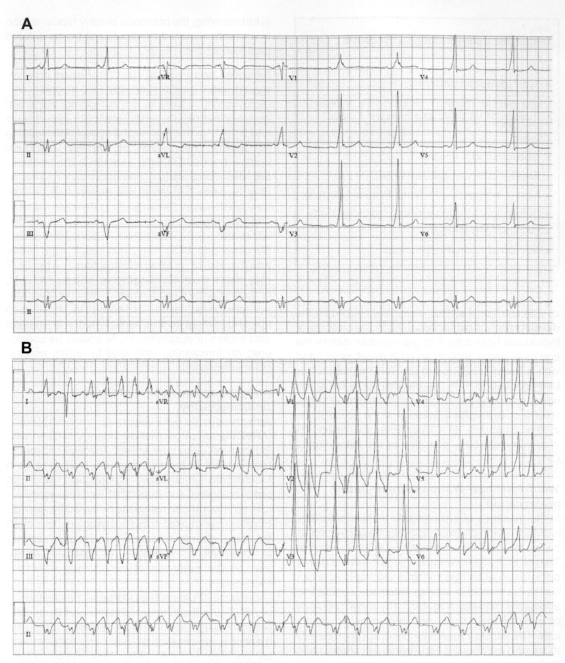

Fig. 5. Twelve-lead ECG from a patient with Wolff-Parkinson-White syndrome. (*A*) Evidence of manifest preexcitation at baseline with short PR interval and slurred onset of QRS (delta wave). (*B*) Atrial fibrillation with rapid ventricular conduction via the accessory pathway in the same patient.

circulatory demands, especially during exertion. The obstruction may occur at any level of the circulatory system, and may be either fixed or dynamic. Fixed obstructive lesions may include valvular or paravalvular lesions such as aortic stenosis, mitral stenosis, and supravalvular and subvalvular webs or ridges. Dynamic lesions may include conditions such as HCM with LVOT

obstruction, or intracardiac tumors such as atrial myxomas. Disease processes that limit LV filling, such as pericardial tamponade, pulmonary hypertension, and pulmonary emboli, may also result in syncope.[1,12] Most mechanical causes of syncope may be identified with a physical assessment and a thorough echocardiographic examination, and are often considered life threatening.

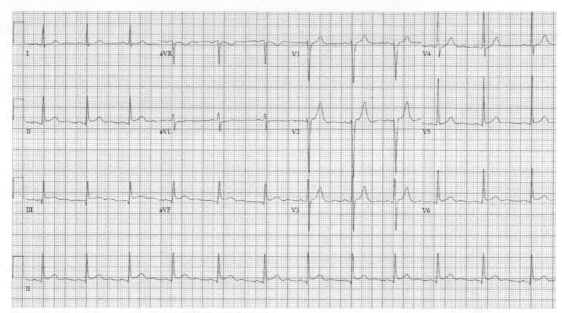

Fig. 6. Early repolarization in the inferolateral leads of a 12-lead ECG obtained from a young individual with recurrent syncope and an otherwise normal cardiac workup. The implications of this are unclear, and other mechanisms of syncope should be sought.

DIAGNOSTIC APPROACH TO IDENTIFYING LIFE-THREATENING CAUSES OF SYNCOPE

A staged approach to the diagnostic workup of syncope has been suggested by several investigators and society guidelines (**Box 5**).[12,51,52] One of the chief objectives in the initial evaluation is to identify individuals at higher risk of adverse outcomes for whom more sophisticated or invasive testing might be required to firmly obtain an etiologic diagnosis. Several risk scores have been developed that synthesize data from the initial evaluation to aid in the identification of individuals at higher risk. Certain risk scores, such as the San

---

Box 4
Diagnostic clues for arrhythmogenic right ventricular cardiomyopathy

Clinical
- ARVC confirmed in a first-degree relative
- Identification of a pathogenic mutation associated with ARVC

Imaging
- Right ventricular enlargement, akinesia, dyskinesia, or aneurysm by echocardiography, angiography, or MRI

Histology
- Myocyte loss with fibrous replacement of the right ventricular free wall myocardium with or without fatty replacement of tissue on endomyocardial biopsy

ECG
- Inverted T waves in right precordial leads (V1, V2, V3) or beyond in individuals older than 14 years
- Epsilon wave in the right precordial leads (V1–V3)
- Late potentials by SAECG

Arrhythmias
- Nonsustained or sustained VT of left bundle branch morphology
- More than 500 ventricular extrasystoles per 24 hours on Holter monitoring

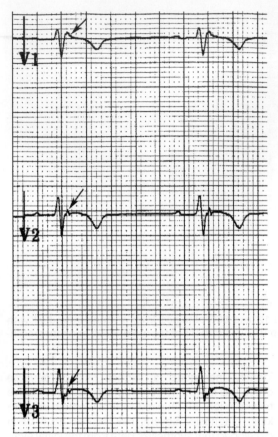

Fig. 7. Epsilon waves (*arrows*) in a patient with arrhythmogenic right ventricular cardiomyopathy.

Francisco Syncope Rule and the OESIL (Osservatorio Epidemiologico sulla Sincope nel Lazio) score, have been validated across several clinical settings (**Table 1**).[53–56] Significant overlap in these risk scores exists, however, and thus the recognition of potentially high-risk features generally suffices in routine clinical practice.

As symptom-rhythm correlation with ECG is vital in making a diagnosis of bradycardia or tachyarrhythmia, further tests including head-up tilt-table testing, electrophysiology (EP) studies, or longer-term monitoring with an implantable loop recorder (ILR) may be indicated. Where possible, efforts should be made to acquire previous ECGs, telemetry strips, and Holter monitoring results, as certain diagnoses may only be intermittently apparent.

Historical Features

A general approach to the patient with syncope is outlined in the article by Benditt and colleagues elsewhere in this issue. Focusing on the recognition of life-threatening causes, a key first step is a careful history focusing on preexisting cardiovascular disease, ventricular arrhythmias, and a history of congestive heart failure (CHF), which have been universally identified as risk markers of cardiac syncope.[53,54,57–59] Incrementally it is crucial to determine the context of syncope, because many of the unusual but life-threatening genetic causes will occur in the context of specific triggers. LQTS and CPVT often involve swimming,

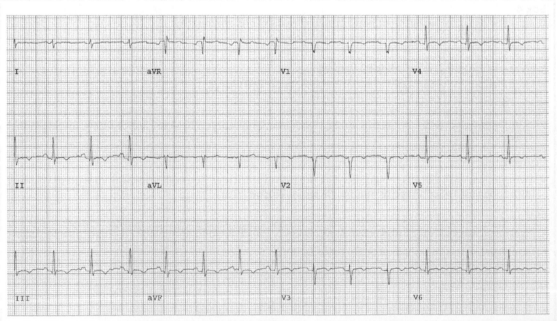

Fig. 8. Diffuse T-wave inversions in anterior precordial leads persisting past V4 in a patient with established arrhythmogenic right ventricular cardiomyopathy.

Box 5
Approach to potentially life-threatening syncope

- Patient profile
  - Older individual
  - History of structural heart disease
- History
  - Syncope history compatible with a cardiac etiology (**Tables 1** and **2**)
  - Family history of SCD or life-threatening causes of syncope
  - Unusual context of syncope
- Physical examination
  - Evidence of heart failure or ventricular dysfunction
  - Murmurs compatible with valvular obstruction
  - Evidence of hypertrophic cardiomyopathy: S4, dynamic LV outflow obstruction
- 12-Lead ECG (see **Box 6**) and ECG monitoring
  - Obtain previous ECGs, telemetry, and Holter recordings where possible
- Echocardiography
- Further investigations if warranted (see **Box 7**)

---

auditory or emotional stimuli, startle, or exercise. These contexts are distinctly unusual in "garden-variety" vasovagal syncope. A family history of syncope, SCD, or suspicious deaths (eg, unexplained drownings, single-vehicular accidents, or presumed heart attacks at a young age) should also raise suspicion for an inherited cause of cardiac syncope.[22] Detailed history taking of the events surrounding the syncopal event is invaluable, often involving the interview of a bystander observer. The presence of dyspnea and chest pain is more often, but not necessarily, found with cardiac syncope.[60,61] The specificity of palpitations for an arrhythmia is questionable, as they may be reported before neurocardiogenic syncope.[11,60] However, a description of an irregularly irregular rhythm before syncope may suggest

a conversion pause following atrial fibrillation.[1] The absence of a significant prodromal period is suggestive of a Stokes-Adams attack or a primary arrhythmia, which has been traditionally attributed to an arrhythmic cause.[62,63] In one study, a prodromal duration of 5 seconds or less was suggestive of an arrhythmia (positive likelihood ratio = 2.4); however, one-third of patients with neurocardiogenic syncope also had a prodrome lasting less than 5 seconds, whereas VT presented with a longer prodromal period.[11]

The context of the syncopal episode is also important. Syncope in the supine position or with exertion has been shown to be associated with cardiac syncope.[58,64,65] Stokes-Adams attacks may occur in any position.[62] Exertional syncope is virtually always an alarming signal that warrants

---

Table 1
Clinical risk factors as identified by syncope risk scores

San Francisco Syncope Rule[53]	OESIL Score[54]	EGSYS Score[58]
Abnormal ECG	Abnormal ECG	Palpitations before syncope
Congestive heart failure	History of cardiovascular disease	Abnormal ECG and/or heart disease
Shortness of breath	Lack of prodrome	Syncope during effort
Hematocrit <30%	Age >65 y	Syncope while supine
Systolic blood pressure <90 mm Hg		Lack of autonomic prodrome
		Lack of predisposing and/or precipitating factors

Table 2
Historical features suggestive of cardiac syncope

Baseline Characteristics	Before Syncope	Syncopal Event	Following Syncope
Prior history of cardiovascular disease	Lack of autonomic prodrome	Supine position	Short duration of symptoms following syncope
Prior history of ventricular arrhythmias	Dyspnea	Exertional syncope	Lack of prolonged fatigue
Prior history of congestive heart failure	Chest pain	Syncope during sleep	
Family history of syncope or cardiac arrest	Palpitations	Syncope with emotional distress	
Unusual context of syncope (exertion, auditory stimulus)	Prodrome <5 s		

urgent specialized assessment. It may occur in individuals with obstruction to ventricular outflow, but may also occur with inheritable conditions such as LQTS, CPVT, and ARVC.[22,32,62,66,67] On the other hand, syncope following cessation of exercise is more likely to be neurocardiogenic. Syncope during sleep or with emotional distress may also be suggestive of a channelopathy such as LQTS or BS.[22,30] The period following the syncopal episode also provides clues as to the underlying etiology. Prolonged fatigue is suggestive of neurocardiogenic syncope, and the lack of prompt resolution of symptoms following syncope makes cardiac syncope much less likely (**Table 2**).[11,61,62]

Physical Examination

A focused cardiovascular physical examination may reveal clues suggesting a cardiac cause for syncope (see **Box 5**). A systolic murmur compatible with severe aortic stenosis provides a putative cause for syncope, as does the systolic murmur of HCM with LVOT obstruction that increases with Valsalva maneuver or squat-to-stand maneuver.[42] A diastolic rumble may suggest significant mitral stenosis or a tumor obstructing LV inflow.

Twelve-Lead ECG

Although the diagnostic yield of the 12-lead ECG is fairly low,[7] an abnormal ECG should automatically raise the prospect of a cardiac cause of syncope. Red flags for either a bradyarrhythmic or tachyarrhythmic cause of syncope should be sought (**Box 6**).[12] Evidence of a malfunctioning pacemaker or defibrillator is rare, but may also be detected on an ECG. Linking the history with the ECG to

evaluate voltage, conduction, and repolarization is crucial when related causes are suspected.

Echocardiography

Although the diagnostic yield of an echocardiogram is low in all-comers presenting with syncope, it continues to play an important role in confirming

Box 6
ECG red flags for worrisome causes of syncope

Bradyarrhythmias
- Persistent sinus bradycardia less than 40 beats/min while awake
- Sinus pauses 3 seconds or more
- Mobitz II atrioventricular block
- Complete heart block or alternating bundle branch block

Tachyarrhythmias
- Documented VT or VF
- Pathologic Q waves
- Evidence of LV hypertrophy
- Abnormal prolongation or shortening of QTc
- Brugada pattern ECG
- Manifest preexcitation
- Epsilon waves, T-wave inversions from V1 to V3

Repolarization Changes
- QT interval, long or short (LQTS, SQTS)
- T-wave inversion in the anterior precordial leads (ARVC)
- ST elevation in the anterior precordial leads (Brugada)

or refuting the presence of structural heart disease in individuals for whom sufficient suspicion exists based on the history or physical examination.[68] It is able to definitively identify mechanical causes of syncope, while also providing the ability to risk stratify individuals based on the LVEF.[12]

SPECIALIZED TESTING MODALITIES USEFUL IN SELECT PATIENTS

If the etiology of cardiac-sounding syncope remains uncertain after initial investigations are complete, further investigations can be pursued to aid in confirming or excluding suspected diagnoses (**Box 7**). These tests are outlined in greater detail in other sections, but are summarized briefly here.

Exercise Stress Testing

Aside from the identification of those with suspected cardiac ischemia, the exercise stress test (ETT) is valuable in the workup of those with life-threatening causes of syncope. It can be used to evaluate exertional syncope potentially caused by obstructive or ischemic sources.[69] The ETT is of diagnostic utility in patients with LQTS, for whom failed shortening of the QT with exercise or in recovery can identify those carrying an LQTS-conferring genetic mutation.[18] In addition, the development of second-degree or third-degree heart block with exercise identifies those with significant infra-Hisian conduction-system disease and a potentially unreliable escape rhythm.[12]

Ambulatory ECG Monitoring

The yield of Holter monitors and external loop recorders in detecting arrhythmic causes of syncope are limited by their relatively short duration of data collection. As a result, their use is largely limited to those with fairly frequent

---

Box 7
Role of further testing modalities for selected patients with worrisome syncope

1. Exercise ECG testing

   a. Investigation of suspected cardiac ischemia, workup of exertional syncope

   b. Confirmation of suspected LQTS, CPVT, or evidence of high-grade AV block

   c. Risk stratification of patients with manifest preexcitation

2. ILR

   a. Provides continuous monitoring for up to 3 years' duration

   b. For symptom-rhythm correlation in patients with infrequent episodes of cardiac-sounding syncope and no readily apparent diagnosis

3. Cardiac MRI

   a. Identification of subtle structural heart disease, myocardial scarring, or myocarditis when ventricular tachyarrhythmias are suspected in an individual with an apparently structurally normal heart

4. Electrophysiologic testing

   a. Investigation of patients with structural heart disease or abnormal ECG with cardiac syncope but not meeting indications for an ICD or pacemaker

   b. Identification of patients with readily inducible VT or conduction-system disease

5. Pharmacologic challenge

   a. Intravenous infusion of epinephrine used to aid in diagnosis of LQTS

   b. Intravenous infusion of procainamide used to aid in diagnosis of BS

6. Head-up tilt table testing

   a. Noninvasive test used to reproduce symptoms of vasovagal or orthostatic syncope

   b. Most useful in patients with an intermediate probability of vasovagal syncope; reproduction of symptoms confirms the diagnosis of vasovagal syncope

7. Signal-averaged ECG

   a. Identification of late potentials resulting from delayed ventricular depolarization associated with myocardial scarring

   b. Mainstream clinical use limited, but may be used to assist in diagnosis of ARVC

events.[7,12] ILRs allow for longer periods of monitoring, as the devices may be implanted for up to 3 years. Patients with a preexisting pacemaker or defibrillator should have their device interrogated to correlate any recorded high ventricular rate events during the time of their symptoms.

Electrophysiologic Testing

The objective of EP testing is to identify the cause of syncope by either the induction of a tachyarrhythmia or the determination of underlying conduction-system disease. As it is difficult to definitively attribute the cause of syncope to arrhythmias induced during the EP study, its use has been reserved largely for cases with evidence of structural heart disease or abnormal ECGs whereby noninvasive testing has failed to establish a firm diagnosis and an ICD is not warranted by the ejection fraction (typically ≤40%).[1]

SUMMARY

The identification of syncopal individuals at increased risk requires a thorough clinical approach including a careful history, physical examination, 12-lead ECG, and an echocardiogram. Awareness of life-threatening causes of syncope should lead the clinician to search for red flags that may raise suspicion for one of these causes. The use of further noninvasive and invasive testing modalities may then be used to confirm the diagnosis. Where possible, involvement of specialist cardiology and cardiac electrophysiology services in such cases will help facilitate the selection of appropriate tests and subsequent therapeutic options.

REFERENCES

1. Angaran P, Klein GJ, Yee R, et al. Syncope. Neurol Clin 2011;29(4):903–25.
2. Kapoor WN, Karpf M, Wieand S, et al. A prospective evaluation and follow-up of patients with syncope. N Engl J Med 1983;309(4):197–204.
3. Soteriades ES, Evans JC, Larson MG, et al. Incidence and prognosis of syncope. N Engl J Med 2002;347(12):878–85.
4. Ganzeboom KS, Mairuhu G, Reitsma JB, et al. Lifetime cumulative incidence of syncope in the general population: a study of 549 Dutch subjects aged 35-60 years. J Cardiovasc Electrophysiol 2006;17(11):1172–6.
5. Kapoor WN. Evaluation and outcome of patients with syncope. Medicine 1990;69(3):160–75.
6. Eagle KA, Black HR, Cook EF, et al. Evaluation of prognostic classifications for patients with syncope. Am J Med 1985;79(4):455–60.
7. Mitro P, Kirsch P, Valocik G, et al. A prospective study of the standardized diagnostic evaluation of syncope. Europace 2011;13(4):566–71.
8. Baron-Esquivias G, Errazquin F, Pedrote A, et al. Long-term outcome of patients with vasovagal syncope. Am Heart J 2004;147(5):883–9.
9. Olshansky B, Poole JE, Johnson G, et al. Syncope predicts the outcome of cardiomyopathy patients: analysis of the SCD-HeFT study. J Am Coll Cardiol 2008;51(13):1277–82.
10. Ungar A, Del Rosso A, Giada F, et al. Early and late outcome of treated patients referred for syncope to emergency department: the EGSYS 2 follow-up study. Eur Heart J 2010;31(16):2021–6.
11. Calkins H, Shyr Y, Frumin H, et al. The value of the clinical history in the differentiation of syncope due to ventricular tachycardia, atrioventricular block, and neurocardiogenic syncope. Am J Med 1995;98(4):365–73.
12. Moya A, Sutton R, Ammirati F, et al. Guidelines for the diagnosis and management of syncope (version 2009). Eur Heart J 2009;30(21):2631–71.
13. Barold SS, Hayes DL. Second-degree atrioventricular block: a reappraisal. Mayo Clin Proc 2001;76(1):44–57.
14. Greenberg H, McMaster P, Dwyer EM Jr. Left ventricular dysfunction after acute myocardial infarction: results of a prospective multicenter study. J Am Coll Cardiol 1984;4(5):867–74.
15. Buxton AE, Lee KL, Hafley GE, et al. Limitations of ejection fraction for prediction of sudden death risk in patients with coronary artery disease: lessons from the MUSTT study. J Am Coll Cardiol 2007;50(12):1150–7.
16. Bokil NJ, Baisden JM, Radford DJ, et al. Molecular genetics of long QT syndrome. Mol Genet Metab 2010;101(1):1–8.
17. Schwartz PJ, Stramba-Badiale M, Crotti L, et al. Prevalence of the congenital long-QT syndrome. Circulation 2009;120(18):1761–7.
18. Sy RW, van der Werf C, Chattha IS, et al. Derivation and validation of a simple exercise-based algorithm for prediction of genetic testing in relatives of LQTS probands. Circulation 2011;124(20):2187–94.
19. Wong JA, Gula LJ, Klein GJ, et al. Utility of treadmill testing in identification and genotype prediction in long-QT syndrome. Circ Arrhythm Electrophysiol 2010;3(2):120–5.
20. Goldenberg I, Moss AJ. Long QT syndrome. J Am Coll Cardiol 2008;51(24):2291–300.
21. Schwartz PJ, Moss AJ, Vincent GM, et al. Diagnostic criteria for the long QT syndrome. An update. Circulation 1993;88(2):782–4.
22. Colman N, Bakker A, Linzer M, et al. Value of history-taking in syncope patients: in whom to suspect long QT syndrome? Europace 2009;11(7):937–43.

23. Priori SG, Cerrone M. Genetic arrhythmias. Ital Heart J 2005;6(3):241–8.

24. Sarkozy A, Brugada P. Sudden cardiac death: what is inside our genes? Can J Cardiol 2005;21(12): 1099–110.

25. Lehnart SE, Ackerman MJ, Benson DW Jr, et al. Inherited arrhythmias: a National Heart, Lung, and Blood Institute and Office of Rare Diseases workshop consensus report about the diagnosis, phenotyping, molecular mechanisms, and therapeutic approaches for primary cardiomyopathies of gene mutations affecting ion channel function. Circulation 2007;116(20):2325–45.

26. Gollob MH, Redpath CJ, Roberts JD. The short QT syndrome: proposed diagnostic criteria. J Am Coll Cardiol 2011;57(7):802–12.

27. Lippi G, Montagnana M, Meschi T, et al. Genetic and clinical aspects of Brugada syndrome: an update. Adv Clin Chem 2012;56:197–208.

28. Nademanee K, Veerakul G, Nimmannit S, et al. Arrhythmogenic marker for the sudden unexplained death syndrome in Thai men. Circulation 1997; 96(8):2595–600.

29. Miyasaka Y, Tsuji H, Yamada K, et al. Prevalence and mortality of the Brugada-type electrocardiogram in one city in Japan. J Am Coll Cardiol 2001; 38(3):771–4.

30. Antzelevitch C, Brugada P, Borggrefe M, et al. Brugada syndrome: report of the second consensus conference: endorsed by the Heart Rhythm Society and the European Heart Rhythm Association. Circulation 2005;111(5):659–70.

31. Sangwatanaroj S, Prechawat S, Sunsaneewitayakul B, et al. New electrocardiographic leads and the procainamide test for the detection of the Brugada sign in sudden unexplained death syndrome survivors and their relatives. Eur Heart J 2001;22(24):2290–6.

32. Priori SG, Napolitano C, Memmi M, et al. Clinical and molecular characterization of patients with catecholaminergic polymorphic ventricular tachycardia. Circulation 2002;106(1):69–74.

33. Sy RW, Gollob MH, Klein GJ, et al. Arrhythmia characterization and long-term outcomes in catecholaminergic polymorphic ventricular tachycardia. Heart Rhythm 2011;8(6):864–71.

34. Napolitano C, Priori SG. Diagnosis and treatment of catecholaminergic polymorphic ventricular tachycardia. Heart Rhythm 2007;4(5):675–8.

35. Klein GJ, Bashore TM, Sellers TD, et al. Ventricular fibrillation in the Wolff-Parkinson-White syndrome. N Engl J Med 1979;301(20):1080–5.

36. Haissaguerre M, Derval N, Sacher F, et al. Sudden cardiac arrest associated with early repolarization. N Engl J Med 2008;358(19):2016–23.

37. Rosso R, Kogan E, Belhassen B, et al. J-point elevation in survivors of primary ventricular fibrillation and matched control subjects: incidence and clinical significance. J Am Coll Cardiol 2008; 52(15):1231–8.

38. Tikkanen JT, Anttonen O, Junttila MJ, et al. Long-term outcome associated with early repolarization on electrocardiography. N Engl J Med 2009; 361(26):2529–37.

39. Stern S. Clinical aspects of the early repolarization syndrome: a 2011 update. Ann Noninvasive Electrocardiol 2011;16(2):192–5.

40. Gersh BJ, Maron BJ, Bonow RO, et al. 2011 ACCF/ AHA guideline for the diagnosis and treatment of hypertrophic cardiomyopathy: executive summary: a report of the American College of Cardiology Foundation/American Heart Association Task Force on Practice Guidelines. Circulation 2011;124(24): 2761–96.

41. Marian AJ. Hypertrophic cardiomyopathy: from genetics to treatment. Eur J Clin Invest 2010;40(4): 360–9.

42. Towbin JA. Hypertrophic cardiomyopathy. Pacing Clin Electrophysiol 2009;32(Suppl 2):S23–31.

43. Basso C, Corrado D, Marcus FI, et al. Arrhythmogenic right ventricular cardiomyopathy. Lancet 2009;373(9671):1289–300.

44. Sen-Chowdhry S, Syrris P, Ward D, et al. Clinical and genetic characterization of families with arrhythmogenic right ventricular dysplasia/cardiomyopathy provides novel insights into patterns of disease expression. Circulation 2007;115(13):1710–20.

45. Corrado D, Fontaine G, Marcus FI, et al. Arrhythmogenic right ventricular dysplasia/cardiomyopathy: need for an international registry. Study Group on Arrhythmogenic Right Ventricular Dysplasia/Cardiomyopathy of the Working Groups on Myocardial and Pericardial Disease and Arrhythmias of the European Society of Cardiology and of the Scientific Council on Cardiomyopathies of the World Heart Federation. Circulation 2000;101(11):E101–6.

46. Marcus FI, McKenna WJ, Sherrill D, et al. Diagnosis of arrhythmogenic right ventricular cardiomyopathy/ dysplasia: proposed modification of the task force criteria. Circulation 2010;121(13):1533–41.

47. Cox MG, Nelen MR, Wilde AA, et al. Activation delay and VT parameters in arrhythmogenic right ventricular dysplasia/cardiomyopathy: toward improvement of diagnostic ECG criteria. J Cardiovasc Electrophysiol 2008;19(8):775–81.

48. Jain R, Dalal D, Daly A, et al. Electrocardiographic features of arrhythmogenic right ventricular dysplasia. Circulation 2009;120(6):477–87.

49. Kamath GS, Zareba W, Delaney J, et al. Value of the signal-averaged electrocardiogram in arrhythmogenic right ventricular cardiomyopathy/dysplasia. Heart Rhythm 2011;8(2):256–62.

50. Fontaine G, Fontaliran F, Hebert JL, et al. Arrhythmogenic right ventricular dysplasia. Annu Rev Med 1999;50:17–35.

51. Krahn AD, Klein GJ, Yee R, et al. The use of monitoring strategies in patients with unexplained syncope—role of the external and implantable loop recorder. Clin Auton Res 2004;14(Suppl 1):55–61.

52. Moya A, Garcia-Civera R, Croci F, et al. Diagnosis, management, and outcomes of patients with syncope and bundle branch block. Eur Heart J 2011;32(12):1535–41.

53. Quinn J, McDermott D, Stiell I, et al. Prospective validation of the San Francisco Syncope Rule to predict patients with serious outcomes. Ann Emerg Med 2006;47(5):448–54.

54. Colivicchi F, Ammirati F, Melina D, et al. Development and prospective validation of a risk stratification system for patients with syncope in the emergency department: the OESIL risk score. Eur Heart J 2003;24(9):811–9.

55. Serrano LA, Hess EP, Bellolio MF, et al. Accuracy and quality of clinical decision rules for syncope in the emergency department: a systematic review and meta-analysis. Ann Emerg Med 2010;56(4):362–373.e1.

56. Saccilotto RT, Nickel CH, Bucher HC, et al. San Francisco Syncope Rule to predict short-term serious outcomes: a systematic review. CMAJ 2011;183(15):E1116–26.

57. Martin TP, Hanusa BH, Kapoor WN. Risk stratification of patients with syncope. Ann Emerg Med 1997;29(4):459–66.

58. Del Rosso A, Ungar A, Maggi R, et al. Clinical predictors of cardiac syncope at initial evaluation in patients referred urgently to a general hospital: the EGSYS score. Heart 2008;94(12):1620–6.

59. Sun BC, Derose SF, Liang LJ, et al. Predictors of 30-day serious events in older patients with syncope. Ann Emerg Med 2009;54(6):769–778.e1–5.

60. Galizia G, Abete P, Mussi C, et al. Role of early symptoms in assessment of syncope in elderly people: results from the Italian group for the study of syncope in the elderly. J Am Geriatr Soc 2009;57(1):18–23.

61. Mitro P, Kirsch P, Valocik G, et al. Clinical history in the diagnosis of the cardiac syncope—the predictive scoring system. Pacing Clin Electrophysiol 2011;34(11):1480–5.

62. Wayne HH. Syncope. Physiological considerations and an analysis of the clinical characteristics in 510 patients. Am J Med 1961;30:418–38.

63. Pomerantz B, O'Rourke RA. The Stokes-Adams syndrome. Am J Med 1969;46(6):941–60.

64. Krahn AD, Healey JS, Simpson CS, et al. Sentinel symptoms in patients with unexplained cardiac arrest: from the cardiac arrest survivors with preserved ejection fraction registry (CASPER). J Cardiovasc Electrophysiol 2012;23(1):60–6.

65. Del Rosso A, Alboni P, Brignole M, et al. Relation of clinical presentation of syncope to the age of patients. Am J Cardiol 2005;96(10):1431–5.

66. Tavora F, Zhang M, Franco M, et al. Distribution of biventricular disease in arrhythmogenic cardiomyopathy: an autopsy study. Hum Pathol 2012;43(4):592–6.

67. Bhonsale A, James CA, Tichnell C, et al. Incidence and predictors of implantable cardioverter-defibrillator therapy in patients with arrhythmogenic right ventricular dysplasia/cardiomyopathy undergoing implantable cardioverter-defibrillator implantation for primary prevention. J Am Coll Cardiol 2011;58(14):1485–96.

68. Recchia D, Barzilai B. Echocardiography in the evaluation of patients with syncope. J Gen Intern Med 1995;10(12):649–55.

69. Linzer M, Yang EH, Estes NA 3rd, et al. Diagnosing syncope. Part 2: unexplained syncope. Clinical Efficacy Assessment Project of the American College of Physicians. Ann Intern Med 1997;127(1):76–86.

Tilt Table Testing and Implantable Loop Recorders for Syncope

Robert Sheldon, MD, PhD

KEYWORDS

• Tilt table tests • Implantable loop recorders • Syncope • Randomized studies • Diagnosis

KEY POINTS

- Tilt table tests have provided important benefits in the field of neurally mediated syncope; however, they have significant limitations.
- Tilt table tests have many significant methodological variables, have not been validated against gold standard populations, are only moderately reproducible, do not provide prognostic predictive power, and have not been shown useful in selecting effective therapies.
- Implantable loop recorders (ILRs) are small, subcutaneous digital recording devices with a lifespan of 2 to 3 years. Randomized studies have established the safety and efficacy of their early application in the diagnosis of syncope.
- About 40% of patients have syncope and a diagnosis its cause while bearing ILRs.
- ILRs have identified 2 populations of older patients with syncope who may benefit from permanent pacing.

INTRODUCTION

Neurally mediated syncope is a common problem. Numerous epidemiologic studies have shown that the lifetime prevalence is over 40%, and many people faint recurrently.[1-3] Not surprisingly, many people who faint seek help. Syncope is responsible for 1% to 6% of emergency room visits and 1% to 3% of hospital admissions, and it is a frequent reason for referral to internists, cardiologists, and neurologists.[4,5] Some causes of syncope are potentially fatal, and, coupled with a limited insight into the symptoms that surround syncope, many physicians are uncertain about how to approach the diagnostic process with both accuracy and efficiency.

The European Society of Cardiology guidelines[4] provide streamlined guidance for the diagnosis of syncope. They are written generally from the perspective of consulting cardiologists and advocate the use of a detailed history early in the diagnostic process. A comprehensive history can provide a wealth of useful information, and structured histories and point scores are useful for the initial, rapid diagnosis of syncope versus epileptic seizures,[6] syncope with a structurally normal heart,[7] and syncope with structural heart disease.[8] They also are useful in risk stratification in the emergency room,[9] and in predicting the likelihood of syncope recurrences.[5]

Many patients, however, continue to provide diagnostic challenges after the initial assessment. Most of these patients require further investigation. An electrocardiogram (ECG) is warranted in all patients, and following this, the 2 most useful diagnostic tools are the tilt table test and the implantable loop recorder (ILR). This article will review both these tools and provide some suggestions on deciding when and which of them to use.

Libin Cardiovascular Institute of Alberta, University of Calgary, 3280 Hospital Drive Northwest, Calgary, Alberta T2N 4N1, Canada
E-mail address: sheldon@ucalgary.ca

Cardiol Clin 31 (2013) 67–74
http://dx.doi.org/10.1016/j.ccl.2012.10.009
0733-8651/13/$ – see front matter © 2013 Elsevier Inc. All rights reserved.

TILT TABLE TESTS
History of Tilt Table Tests

Tilt table tests were initially used as tools to study compensatory responses to orthostatic stress, and their ability to induce syncope was recognized in the middle of the 20th century by US Air Force clinical investigators. This was prompted by studies that showed that 25% of US Air Force personnel had a history of syncope.[4] Somewhat later, civilian physicians, faced with the diagnostic challenge of syncope and the ability of tilt table tests to induce vasovagal syncope, developed them as clinical tools. Tilt table tests now are widely used for diagnosing syncope, and have also been used as tools for physiologic studies, predicting outcome, and selecting therapies.

Types of Tilt Table Tests

The core of tilt table testing is passive head-upright tilt for 20 to 60 minutes, until hypotension, bradycardia, presyncope, or syncope ensues, or until the test ends (**Box 1**). Prolonged orthostatic stress may be coupled with intravenous isoproterenol, sublingual nitrates, or intravenous clomipramine[10] to induce an endpoint. Nitrates are given to increase venodilation; isoproterenol is given to mimic the catecholamine response to stress, and clomipramine is given to increase intracranial serotonin, which is postulated to be a neurotransmitter central to the reflex. Combinations of these variables led to a large number of individual tilt table test protocols, each with its own reported accuracy.[11] On average, positive response in patients with prior syncope occurs in 49% of passive tests and 66% of tests with an additional provocative factor. They have been used in diagnostic studies in populations such as those with neurally mediated syncope, syncope in the setting of structural heart disease, loss of consciousness that might be due to syncope or epilepsy, postural orthostatic tachycardia, and autonomic neuropathy.[4] They have been used as

---

Box 1
How are tilt table tests performed?

Patients are awake and alert and gently restrained on a table capable of head-up tilt

Table pivoted upwards at 60° to 80°

Intravenous isoproterenol or clomipramine or sublingual nitrates may be included

Generally last up to 45 minutes

End points: presyncope or syncop, and hypotension and/or bradycardia

---

entry criteria in observational studies and clinical trials, mechanistic studies of the vasovagal reflex, and in drug studies, and they have been proposed to be useful for selecting efficacious treatment. However, their true usefulness has not been validated.

Tilt table tests have made several significant contributions. They have made the informed care of syncope patients more accessible and less daunting, and by their ability to induce syncope under controlled conditions have reassured many patients about the diagnosis and provided a measure of comfort to physicians. They have provided the inclusion criteria for diagnostic and long-term observational studies and randomized clinical trials. Tilt table tests have been used as platforms for physiologic studies and pilot treatment studies. However, there are limitations to the use and interpretation of studies based on or including tilt table tests.

Test Accuracy

The central problem is that there is not a good evidence-based clinical definition of a syndrome of neurally mediated syncope. In essence, it is a syndrome defined by a test, rather than a test that diagnoses a syndrome. There is a lack of the validation of tilt table testing against populations with defined causes of syncope.[12] This causes problems with defining or knowing the sensitivity of tilt table tests, raising the issue of whether patients with negative tests have a different syndrome. This is a genuine concern. Patients with negative and positive tests have similar symptoms,[7] similar symptom burdens,[7] similar clinical outcomes in the 3 years following the tilt table test,[13] and have ties between symptoms and outcomes.[13–15] These results suggest that a significant number of patients with neurally mediated syncope may have falsely negative tilt table tests. Therefore, a positive tilt table test may be an epiphenomenon associated with neurally mediated syncope, rather than a core feature. Lelonek and colleagues[16] reported that a single nucleotide polymorphism in a G protein is associated with negative tilt table tests in syncope patients.

Studies of the specificity of tilt table tests are equally difficult to interpret. Numerous studies have reported that the first lifetime syncopal spell can occur at any age, and the lifetime prevalence is at least 20% to 40%.[1–3] It is not known how many control subjects are simply people who have not yet fainted but will at some later time. If tilt table tests identify people predisposed to fainting, then populations of younger control subjects will appear to have more falsely positive tilt

Years),[41] which directly tests whether empirical pacing or therapy targeted by ILR findings provides the best overall outcome in these patients.

The final subgroup of 35 patients had syncope and structural heart disease due to either coronary artery disease or idiopathic dilated cardiomyopathy.[37] The mean LVEF was 47%, and only 6% of patients had an LVEF less than 30%. All had had a negative conventional invasive electrophysiologic study. The patients had a mean follow-up of only 6 months, with a maximum of 19 months. During this time, 6 patients had syncope, and none was due to a VT. Another 6 patients had presyncope, and again none was due to a VT.

Finally, the results of ISSUE 1 led to a proposed scheme for classifying ILR findings during syncope. The intent was to help guide future therapy by diagnosing the cause of syncope from ECG findings alone.[42] The ISSUE 1 reports provided fundamental insights into the mechanism of syncope in a variety of settings, and laid the groundwork for further studies by the ISSUE group. Generally, the investigators proposed that syncope due to cardiac arrhythmias could be diagnosed when there was a symptom-rhythm correlation with tachyarrhythmias, or with abrupt atrioventricular block. Gradually progressive sinus bradycardia that might end with asystole or atrioventricular block was deemed to be due to reflex syncope, such as vasovagal syncope. Lesser changes in heart rate, or sinus tachycardia, were defined as uncertain. This classification resonates with what is known about the vasovagal reflex, but the classification would benefit from outcomes validation.

ISSUE 2 and Guided Therapy

The ISSUE 2 study extended the findings of ISSUE 1 and addressed whether the ILR could be used safely to guide therapy.[36] Three hundred ninety-two subjects with recurrent syncope in the preceding 2 years were enrolled, and all received an ILR. The patients had a mean age of 67 years and were included if other causes of syncope were reasonably excluded and if neurally mediated syncope was suspected. After a median follow-up of 9 months, 103 patients had syncope recurrences. A total of 53 had asystole during syncope, and most subsequently received a dual chamber. Their subsequent course was compared with patients who did not receive pacemaker therapy. Pacing was associated with a relative risk reduction of 80%, and from this it seemed likely that a strategy of pacing guided by ILR findings was both safe and efficacious.

There were residual concerns among the ISSUE investigators and others. The patients were selected as much by excluding other causes as by definite diagnosis of neurally mediated syncope, and other causes of bradycardic syncope exist in older patients.[41,43] The patients were much older than those seen in North America. Finally, comparison of the Vasovagal Pacemaker Studies demonstrated the potential for a very large placebo effect in open-label syncope studies.[32,44,45] To address the latter concern, the investigators undertook ISSUE 3.[46]

ISSUE 3 and Guided Therapy

The structure of ISSUE 3[46] was generally like ISSUE 2, but the final phase involved a double-blind trial of permanent pacing in eligible patients. In this international study, 511 patients with a mean age 63 years and recent frequently recurrent syncope received an ILR.[39] Of these, 89 patients had syncope associated with a prolonged pause, or a long nonsyncopal pause. Subsequently, 77 were randomized to a pacemaker either activated or not, and pacing caused a 32% absolute reduction in the likelihood of a patient having a first faint, and 25% of patients continued to faint despite pacing. For every 100 patients who embarked on an ILR-directed strategy, 17 received pacemakers. Of the paced patients, over the first 2 years, 7 patients would not have fainted without pacing; 6 patients were prevented from fainting, and 4 patients continued to faint. Although an ILR-guided approach does have a statistically significant benefit, only 6 in 100 patients will benefit.

Health Economics and the ILR

There is good evidence that that the ILR provides a diagnosis in a large minority of patients during the lifetime of single ILR. Health care administrators, however, are very interested in the cost utility of ILRs, and whether this information comes at a tolerable cost. The cost was addressed by 2 small randomized trials.

The RAST (Randomized Assessment of Syncope Trial) was reported by Krahn and colleagues[47] in 2003.[48] Sixty patients (mean age 66 years) with syncope and preserved left ventricular function were randomized evenly to early use of an ILR or to conventional assessment with tilt table testing, external loop recorders, and invasive electrophysiologic study. The ILR strategy was diagnostically superior; 14 of 30 ILR subjects received a diagnosis compared with only 6 of 30 subjects with a conventional approach. Overall, a strategy of monitoring followed by tilt table testing and EP testing was associated with a diagnostic yield of 50%, at a cost of $2937 per patient and $5875 per diagnosis. Conventional testing followed by monitoring was associated with an eventual diagnostic yield of

Table 1
EHRA indications for ILRs in patients with syncope

Recommendation	Strength of Recommendation and Level of Evidence
In an early phase of evaluation of patients with recurrent syncope of uncertain origin who have absence of high-risk criteria that require immediate hospitalization or intensive evaluation, and a likely recurrence within battery longevity of the device	Class 1, level A
In high-risk patients in whom a comprehensive evaluation did not demonstrate a cause of syncope or lead to specific treatment	Class 1, level B
To assess the contribution of bradycardia before embarking on cardiac pacing in patients with suspected or certain neurally mediated syncope presenting with frequent or traumatic syncopal episodes	Class 2A, level B
In patients with T-LOC of uncertain syncopal origin to definitely exclude an arrhythmic mechanism	Class 2B, level C

47%, at a greater costs of $3683 per patient and $7891 per diagnosis.

The Eastbourne Syncope Assessment Study (EASYAS) randomized 201 older syncope patients with mean age 74 years to receive an ILR or undergo conventional investigation after early assessment.[49] They were followed for a minimum of 6 months and up to 18 months; as with RAST, the ILR strategy was diagnostically superior. Thirty-four of 103 ILR subjects received a diagnosis compared with only 4 of 98 subjects with a conventional approach. Of the 34 diagnoses made by ILR, 16 were vasovagal syncope, and 3 were hyperventilation. ILR patients had fewer postrandomization investigations and fewer hospital days, resulting in a saving of costs, £406 versus £1210 (mean difference £809). This meant that 60% of the price of the device was recovered. There was no difference in the number of subsequent syncopal spells, mortality, or quality of life.

Although early use of the ILR appears to provide a diagnosis at a reasonable cost, there is as yet no evidence that on an intent-to-insert basis it improves outcome. Much of this is may be due to the lack of effective treatments for most patients with neurally mediated syncope. Nonetheless there is now compelling evidence that early use of ILRs provides more and earlier diagnoses than conventional investigations.

European Heart Rhythm Association Guidelines

The European Heart Rhythm Association (EHRA) issued guidelines for the indications for ILRs in the assessment of syncope.[34] These were informed by the efficacy, safety, and cost utility demonstrated in studies of ILRs for syncope, particularly the EASYAS[49] and RAST[47] studies.

Essentially, the guidelines recommend the early use of ILRs in patients in the middle zone of diagnosis and risk (**Table 1**). They should not be used in low-risk patients, unless they are diagnostic or therapeutic conundrums. Similarly, they should not be used in patients who otherwise have a high risk of adverse outcomes, such as patients with syncope and an indication for implantable cardioverter-defibrillator insertion.

SUMMARY

There now is ample evidence for the roles of tilt table tests and ILRs in the evaluation of syncope.[4,34] The following is a very simplistic approach, but it should suffice in busy cardiology and internal medicine clinics.

Age is the first consideration. Almost all young patients who faint have vasovagal syncope, and this can be teased out and confirmed in most cases with a careful history. Diagnostic scores can serve as memory aids for the main criteria, and as rapid screening tools. The most satisfying approach is to combine knowledge of the physiology of vasovagal syncope with its diagnostic points. Tilt table tests and ILRs should be used with great caution. The concerns are that with a very high probability of vasovagal syncope, negative tilt table tests are likely to be falsely negative,[50] and most vasovagal syncope in younger patients may not be associated with bradycardia. Therefore in younger patients, both tests may be misleading: tilt table tests because of false negatives, and ILRs because only sinus rhythm may be seen.

In older patients (age 50 is a reasonable definition of older), the situation is quite different for several reasons. The history is less sensitive for vasovagal syncope for older patients,[51,52] and tilt table tests are less sensitive but probably more specific. There are numerous competing diagnoses; the risk of potentially fatal causes and comorbidities rises,[53] and at least 2 types of recently understood brady-cardias (neurally mediated syncope and adenosine triphosphate-sensitive heart block) exist. These bradycardias can be treated with permanent pacing.[39,43,54] In older patients (and if the history fails to provide a diagnosis with a high degree of comfort) both options are reasonable. Tilt table tests can be used to establish a diagnosis of vasovagal syncope, and ILRs are a reasonable first investigation. They will detect asymptomatic but relevant arrhythmias, and establish whether patients with vasovagal syncope are candidates for permanent pacing. They should not be used if patients are at high risk of life-threatening arrhythmias, because empirical treatment with defibrillators is proven therapy. The implantable cardioverter-defibrillators may not prevent vasodepressor syncope, but they do prevent death.

REFERENCES

1. Ganzeboom KS, Colman N, Reitsma JB, et al. Prevalence and triggers of syncope in medical students. Am J Cardiol 2003;91:1006–8.
2. Ganzeboom KS, Mairuhu G, Reitsma JB, et al. Lifetime cumulative incidence of syncope in the general population: a study of 549 Dutch subjects aged 35–60 years. J Cardiovasc Electrophysiol 2006;17:1172–6.
3. Serletis A, Rose S, Sheldon AG, et al. Vasovagal syncope in medical students and their first-degree relatives. Eur Heart J 2006;27:1965–70.
4. Moya A, Sutton R, Ammirati F, et al. Guidelines for the diagnosis and management of syncope (version 2009): the Task Force for the Diagnosis and Management of Syncope of the European Society of Cardiology (ESC). Eur Heart J 2009;30:2631–71.
5. Sheldon RS, Morillo CA, Krahn AD, et al. Standardized approaches to the investigation of syncope: Canadian Cardiovascular Society position paper. Can J Cardiol 2011;27:246–53.
6. Sheldon R, Rose S, Ritchie D, et al. Historical criteria that distinguish syncope from seizures. J Am Coll Cardiol 2002;40:142–8.
7. Sheldon R, Rose S, Connolly S, et al. Diagnostic criteria for vasovagal syncope based on a quantitative history. Eur Heart J 2006;27:344–50.
8. Sheldon R, Hersi A, Ritchie D, et al. Syncope and structural heart disease: historical criteria for vasovagal syncope and ventricular tachycardia. J Cardiovasc Electrophysiol 2010;21:1358–64.
9. Sumner GL, Rose MS, Koshman ML, et al. Recent history of vasovagal syncope in a young, referral-based population is a stronger predictor of recurrent syncope than lifetime syncope burden. J Cardiovasc Electrophysiol 2010;21:1375–80.
10. Theodorakis GN, Markianos M, Zarvalis E, et al. Provocation of neurocardiogenic syncope by clomipramine administration during the head-up tilt test in vasovagal syndrome. J Am Coll Cardiol 2000;36:174–8.
11. Delepine S, Prunier F, Leftheriotis G, et al. Comparison between isoproterenol and nitroglycerin sensitized head-upright tilt in patients with unexplained syncope and negative or positive passive head-up tilt response. Am J Cardiol 2002;90:488–91.
12. Agarwal R, Yadave RD, Bhargava B, et al. Head-Up Tilt Test (HUTT) in patients with episodic bradycardia and hypotension following percutaneous coronary interventions. J Invasive Cardiol 1997;9:601–3.
13. Sheldon R, Rose S, Koshman ML. Comparison of patients with syncope of unknown cause having negative or positive tilt-table tests. Am J Cardiol 1997;80:581–5.
14. Grimm W, Degenhardt M, Hoffman J, et al. Syncope recurrence can better be predicted by history than by head-up tilt testing in untreated patients with suspected neurally mediated syncope. Eur Heart J 1997;18:1465–9.
15. Moya A, Brignole M, Menozzi C, et al. Mechanism of syncope in patients with isolated syncope and in patients with tilt-positive syncope. Circulation 2001; 104:1261–7.
16. Lelonek M, Pietrucha T, Matyjaszczyk M, et al. A novel approach to syncopal patients: association analysis of polymorphisms in G-protein genes and tilt outcome. Europace 2009;11:89–93.
17. McIntosh SJ, Lawson J, Kenny RA. Intravenous cannulation alters the specificity of head-up tilt testing for vasovagal syncope in elderly patients. Age Ageing 1994;23:317–9.
18. Sheldon R, Koshman ML. A randomized study of tilt test angle in patients with undiagnosed syncope. Can J Cardiol 2001;17:1051–7.
19. Natale A, Akhtar M, Jazayeri M, et al. Provocation of hypotension during head-up tilt testing in subjects with no history of syncope or presyncope. Circulation 1995;92:54–8.
20. Sheldon R, Killam S. Methodology of isoproterenol-tilt table testing in patients with syncope. J Am Coll Cardiol 1992;19:773–9.
21. Morillo CA, Klein GJ, Zandri S, et al. Diagnostic accuracy of a low-dose isoproterenol head-up tilt protocol. Am Heart J 1995;129:901–6.
22. Burklow TR, Moak JP, Bailey JJ, et al. Neurally mediated cardiac syncope: autonomic modulation after normal saline infusion. J Am Coll Cardiol 1999;33:2059–66.
23. El-Sayed H, Hainsworth R. Salt supplement increases plasma volume and orthostatic tolerance in patients with unexplained syncope. Heart 1996;75:134–40.
24. Mangru NN, Young ML, Mas MS, et al. Usefulness of tilt table test with normal saline infusion in management of neurocardiac syncope in children. Am Heart J 1996; 131:953–5.

25. Bloomfield D, Maurer M, Bigger JT. Effects of age on outcome of tilt table testing. Am J Cardiol 1999;83:1055–8.

26. Sheldon R. Effects of aging on responses to isoproterenol tilt-table testing in patients with syncope. Am J Cardiol 1994;74:459–63.

27. Sheldon R, Sexton E, Koshman ML. Usefulness of clinical factors in predicting outcomes of passive tilt tests in patients with syncope. Am J Cardiol 2000;85:360–4.

28. Sheldon R, Splawinski J, Killam S. Reproducibility of isoproterenol tilt-table tests in patients with syncope. Am J Cardiol 1992;69:1300–5.

29. Sheldon R, Connolly S, Rose S, et al. Prevention of Syncope Trial (POST): a randomized, placebo-controlled study of metoprolol in the prevention of vasovagal syncope. Circulation 2006;113:1164–70.

30. Raj SR, Koshman ML, Sheldon RS. Outcome of patients with dual-chamber pacemakers implanted for the prevention of neurally mediated syncope. Am J Cardiol 2003;91:565–9.

31. Petersen ME, Chamberlain-Webber R, Fitzpatrick AP, et al. Permanent pacing for cardioinhibitory malignant vasovagal syndrome. Br Heart J 1994;71:274–81.

32. Sud S, Massel D, Klein GJ, et al. The expectation effect and cardiac pacing for refractory vasovagal syncope. Am J Med 2007;120:54–62.

33. Parry SW, Matthews IG. Implantable loop recorders in the investigation of unexplained syncope: a state of the art review. Heart 2010;96:1611–6.

34. Brignole M, Vardas P, Hoffman E, et al. Indications for the use of diagnostic implantable and external ECG loop recorders. Europace 2009;11:671–87.

35. Krahn AD, Klein GJ, Norris C, et al. The etiology of syncope in patients with negative tilt table and electrophysiological testing. Circulation 1995;92:1819–24.

36. Brignole M, Sutton R, Menozzi C, et al. Early application of an implantable loop recorder allows effective specific therapy in patients with recurrent suspected neurally mediated syncope. Eur Heart J 2006;27:1085–92.

37. Menozzi C, Brignole M, Garcia-Civera R, et al. Mechanism of syncope in patients with heart disease and negative electrophysiologic test. Circulation 2002;105:2741–5.

38. Edvardsson N, Frykman V, van Mechelen R, et al. Use of an implantable loop recorder to increase the diagnostic yield in unexplained syncope: results from the PICTURE registry. Europace 2011;13:262–9.

39. Brignole M, Menozzi C, Moya A, et al. Pacemaker therapy in patients with neurally mediated syncope and documented asystole: third international study on syncope of uncertain etiology (ISSUE-3): a randomized trial. Circulation 2012;125:2566–71.

40. Brignole M, Menozzi C, Moya A, et al. Mechanism of syncope in patients with bundle branch block and negative electrophysiological test. Circulation 2001;104(17):2045–50.

41. Krahn AD, Morillo CA, Kus T, et al. Empiric pacemaker compared with a monitoring strategy in patients with syncope and bifascicular conduction block–rationale and design of the syncope: pacing or recording in the later years (SPRITELY) study. Europace 2012;14:1044–8.

42. Brignole M, Moya A, Menozzi C, et al. Proposed electrocardiographic classification of spontaneous syncope documented by an implantable loop recorder. Europace 2005;7:14–8.

43. Brignole M, Deharo JC, De Roy L, et al. Syncope due to idiopathic paroxysmal atrioventricular block: long-term follow-up of a distinct form of atrioventricular block. J Am Coll Cardiol 2011;58:167–73.

44. Connolly SJ, Sheldon R, Thorpe KE, et al. Pacemaker therapy for prevention of syncope in patients with recurrent severe vasovagal syncope: second vasovagal pacemaker study (VPS II): a randomized trial. J Am Med Assoc 2003;289:2224–9.

45. Connolly SJ, Sheldon R, Roberts RS, et al. The North American Vasovagal Pacemaker Study (VPS). A randomized trial of permanent cardiac pacing for the prevention of vasovagal syncope. J Am Coll Cardiol 1999;33:16–20.

46. Brignole M. International study on syncope of uncertain aetiology 3 (ISSUE 3): pacemaker therapy for patients with asystolic neutrally mediated syncope: rationale and study design. Europace 2007;9:25–30.

47. Krahn AD, Klein GJ, Yee R, et al. Cost implications of testing strategy in patients with syncope: randomized assessment of syncope trial. J Am Coll Cardiol 2003;42:495–501.

48. Hoch JS, Rockx MA, Krahn AD. Using the net benefit regression framework to construct cost-effectiveness acceptability curves: an example using data from a trial of external loop recorders versus Holter monitoring for ambulatory monitoring of "community acquired" syncope. BMC Health Serv Res 2006;6:68.

49. Farwell DJ, Freemantle N, Sulke AN. Use of implantable loop recorders in the diagnosis and management of syncope. Eur Heart J 2004;25:1257–63.

50. Sheldon R. Tilt testing for syncope: a reappraisal. Curr Opin Cardiol 2005;20:38–41.

51. Rose MS, Sheldon RS, Ritchie D, et al. Calgary syncope symptom score preserves sensitivity for cardiac syncope in aging patients. Heart Rhythm 2010;7:S426.

52. Galizia G, Abete P, Mussi C, et al. Role of early symptoms in assessment of syncope in elderly people: results from the Italian group for the study of syncope in the elderly. J Am Geriatr Soc 2009;57:18–23.

53. Sun BC, Hoffman JR, Mangione CM, et al. Older age predicts short-term, serious events after syncope. J Am Geriatr Soc 2007;55:907–12.

54. Flammang D, Church TR, De Roy L, et al. Treatment of unexplained syncope: a multicenter, randomized trial of cardiac pacing guided by adenosine 5'-triphosphate testing. Circulation 2012;125:31–6.

Vasovagal Syncope
New Physiologic Insights

D.L. Jardine, BSc, MBChB, DCH, FRACP, MD

KEYWORDS

- Vasovagal syncope • Neurocardiogenic syncope • Neurally mediated syncope reflex syncope
- Sympathetic nervous system • Vagus nerve • Microneurography

KEY POINTS

- Vasovagal syncope (VVS) is considered to be reflex in etiology because it is characterized by a transient loss of neural control of circulation; however, the exact anatomic and physiologic nature of this reflex remains uncertain.
- Most patients with recurrent VVS have normal baseline sympathohemodynamics and arterial baroreflex function. After an appropriate adjustment to orthostasis, patients subsequently experience a gradual decrease in blood pressure (BP) for a few minutes.
- In some, the decrease in BP is secondary to decreased cardiac output, while in others it is secondary to simultaneously decreased cardiac output and vasodilatation.
- After a variable time, all patients enter terminal vasodilatation, the mechanism for which may be splanchnic blood pooling, thoracic hypovolemia, and increased ventilation, which in turn may decrease cerebral autoregulation and override the baroreflexes.
- Terminal vasodilatation is usually associated with sympathetic withdrawal and a more rapid decrease in BP followed by bradycardia; syncope occurs secondary to decreased cerebral perfusion as a consequence of this.
- Recovery is immediate on restoration of venous return but may be prolonged in some patients.

INTRODUCTION

The clinician recognizes 3 major triggers for VVS (see **Box 1** for synonyms for VVS):

- Central (in response to emotional stimuli)
- Postural (associated with upright position)
- Situational (in response to specific stimuli)[1,2]

Examples of these triggers include

- Fainting in response to blood–injection–injury phobia (central)
- Fainting during school assembly or while waiting in the checkout queue (postural)
- Micturition syncope (situational)

Postural VVS is by far the most common type and is more likely to occur in ambient heat, while standing after exercise, during a febrile illness, or after drinking a glass of wine in a crowded room. This condition should not be confused with the term "orthostatic syncope," which is usually secondary to initial orthostatic hypotension in the first 30 seconds of standing up, sustained postural hypotension in elderly patients with autonomic failure, or a side-effect of drug treatment.[3] Orthostatic syncope is not discussed further here because its cause is not considered to be primarily vasovagal.

VVS is considered to be reflex in etiology because it is characterized by a transient loss of neural control of circulation.[4] However, the exact anatomic and physiologic nature of this reflex remains uncertain. How and why BP should suddenly decrease in response to prolonged standing or the sight of blood is one of life's great mysteries (**Fig. 1**).

Department of General Medicine, Christchurch Hospital, Private Bag, Riccarton Avenue, Christchurch, New Zealand
E-mail address: david.jardine@cdhb.govt.nz

Cardiol Clin 31 (2013) 75–87
http://dx.doi.org/10.1016/j.ccl.2012.10.010
0733-8651/13/$ – see front matter © 2013 Elsevier Inc. All rights reserved.

HISTORICAL OBJECTIONS TO "THE REFLEX"

The afferent pathway remains uncertain because, for obvious reasons, no human recordings of baroreceptor signals during syncope have been made.

The proposed afferent pathway for VVS has only been properly demonstrated in cats.[5,6] It consists of paradoxic impulses from a hypercontractile, empty left ventricle, which are conducted by unmyelinated vagal afferents to the brain stem. The efferent response is transient vagal stimulation of the heart and widespread sympathetic withdrawal.[7-9] "Applying this reflex to the human requires several leaps of faith" however you could say "applying this reflex to the human requires

several assumptions". First, one has to consider the relevance of this feline reflex, recorded under general anesthesia and major instrumentation, to the conscious human, with the knowledge that animals do not faint.[10] Second, there is good evidence to suggest that humans can faint after cardiac transplantation, when the heart has undergone major efferent and afferent denervation.[11,12] Third, it seems unlikely that this reflex is the main mechanism when the stimulus is central (eg, blood–injection–injury phobia), which may occur in the supine position when the heart is not empty.[13] Finally, echocardiography during tilt has not consistently demonstrated decreased left ventricular size or increased contractility during presyncope, so it is uncertain as to whether there is a "ventricular substrate" for the proposed paradoxic afferent discharge.[14-16]

Therefore, from the outset, although VVS is classified as a form of "reflex syncope," in the human, knowledge of the afferent pathway is limited, and so one cannot be sure that it involves only single reflex.[17] However, a lot has been learnt about the proposed efferent pathways and their effects on the heart and blood vessels during syncope induced in the laboratory.

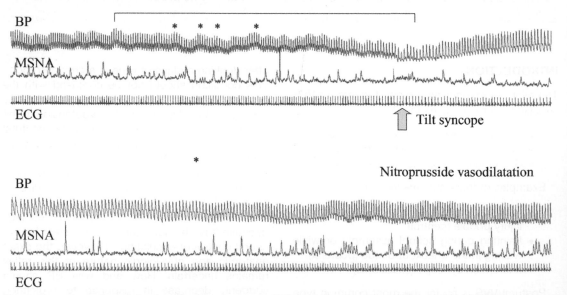

Fig. 1. Two-minute-length tracings for blood pressure (BP), muscle nerve sympathetic activity (MSNA), and heart rate (electrocardiograph [ECG]) during an episode of tilt-induced syncope (*top panel*) and vasodilatation after 150 μg nitroprusside injection (*bottom panel*) in the same patient. The top panel shows blood pressure decreasing rapidly (mean BP from 93 to 68 mm Hg) during the last minute before syncope (*bracket*). During the same time, heart rate decreases (from 121 to 94 bpm). MSNA bursts decrease in frequency (from 37 to 28 bursts/min) and size (from 194% to 107% baseline). Note that in addition to decreasing, the blood pressure is oscillating, typical examples denoted by *asterisk* (cycle length approximately 8 heart beats or 0.25 Hz). The bottom panel shows blood pressure decreasing by a similar magnitude but with less oscillation and an increasing heart rate. MSNA burst frequency and burst size are also steadily increasing throughout.

CONTINUOUS MONITORING IN THE LABORATORY: THE ADVENT OF NONINVASIVE TECHNIQUES AND MICRONEUROGRAPHY

Head-up tilt and lower-body negative pressure (LBNP) studies and continuous monitoring of BP, heart rate (HR), and muscle sympathetic nerve activity (MSNA) have demonstrated a typical sequence of events preceding syncope. This sequence has been clarified over the past 15 years with the introduction of noninvasive measures for monitoring beat-to-beat BP and stroke volume (derived by a computer algorithm) from the arterial waveform.[18] Data demonstrate that, for example, photoplethysmographic estimation of BP from the finger is very similar to that from a brachial artery catheter, even when BP is changing rapidly.[19] The derived values for stroke volume, cardiac output, and total peripheral resistance are used only for assessing trends, not absolute values.[20] Nevertheless, this represents a significant advance from earlier studies of cardiac output, which required intermittent dye injection or thermodilution, allowing only infrequent measurements during presyncope.[21–24]

Since the first human recording of efferent MSNA was reported in 1968, continuous monitoring of MSNA, using the microneurographic technique has become widespread.[25] Several groups have reported MSNA recordings in patient series during VVS induced by tilt, LBNP, and pharmaceutical challenge.[26–30] It is generally accepted that this method gives a dynamic record of adrenergic nerve activity directed to blood vessels.[31,32] However, one must also remember that what is measured here is sympathetic activity directed to the skeletal muscle. During orthostasis, total peripheral resistance is increased mainly by vasoconstriction in the splanchnic and renal vascular beds and, to a lesser extent, in the skin and skeletal muscle; therefore, only part of the sympathoconstrictor response is measured, and it may not be the right part.[25,33,34] Nevertheless, skeletal muscle receives 20% of the total cardiac output at rest, and therefore, any change in vasoconstrictor tone here is likely to have some effect on total peripheral resistance.

Furthermore, during orthostasis, the baroreflex mechanisms decrease blood flow to the skeletal muscle and splanchnic and renal vascular beds by a similar magnitude (about 40%).[35] Therefore, during tilt, and tilt-induced syncope, some changes in the total peripheral resistance may be controlled by MSNA, but splanchnic sympathetic activity is likely more important.[34,35] This fact needs to be taken into account whenever the relationship between MSNA and total peripheral resistance is considered. The simultaneous recording of continuous total peripheral resistance with MSNA is currently the most convenient but not the ideal method for dissecting out different hypotensive mechanisms operating during tilt.[31] Finally, the sequence of events recorded in the laboratory during tilt-induced syncope may not replicate what happens during an "ambulatory" faint (**Fig. 2**).[36,37]

THE SEQUENCE OF EVENTS ACCOMPANYING LABORATORY-INDUCED SYNCOPE
Baseline and Early Tilt

Patients with recurrent syncope generally have normal sympathohemodynamic indices at rest, although there may be a subgroup with resting hypotension, low levels of MSNA, and postural tachycardia.[38] Similarly, in most patients and controls, BP is maintained during the first few minutes of head-up tilt by baroreflex-mediated vasoconstriction: cardiac output and stroke volume usually decrease, while HR, total peripheral resistance, and MSNA increase.[32,39] Traditionally, baroreflexes have been studied by assessing HR responses to changes in systolic BP and sympathoconstrictor responses to both central hypovolemia (low-pressure cardiopulmonary baroreceptors) and hypotension (arterial baroreceptors). This assessment has been done over large pressure ramps (using LBNP, the Valsalva maneuver, neck suction, and drug infusions) and also over small spontaneous pressure fluctuations using spectral analysis and the sequence method.[40]

As stated earlier, it is thought that in humans, BP in the upright position is maintained primarily by vasoconstriction of the skeletal muscle, skin, splanchnic vessels, and renal vessels. Rowell and colleagues[34,35] used forearm plethysmography and dye infusion techniques to demonstrate that at low levels of negative pressure, cardiopulmonary baroreflexes mediated vasoconstriction in the skeletal muscle and skin, whereas at higher levels, carotid and aortic arterial baroreflexes mediated vasoconstriction in the splanchnic and renal vessels. There is clearly some overlap in function between these mechanisms. For example, the carotid baroreceptors are able to respond to changes in central blood volume before mean BP starts to decrease and, by nature of their position above the heart, may sense changes in stroke volume and pulse pressure.[41–43] Because VVS is regarded by most clinicians as a normal physiologic variant, it seems unlikely that all patients with recurrent syncope have

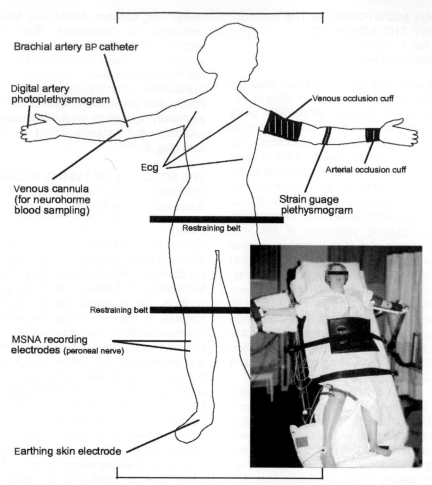

Fig. 2. An example of the recording apparatus for monitoring tilt-induced syncope. The patient is in the head-up 70° position. Most systems do not include the brachial artery catheter, so the arm can be flexed with the finger cuff held in a sling at heart level. Respiration can be measured by thoracic plethysmography indirectly via the electrocardiograph leads or by using a strain gauge. MSNA recordings are taken from the peroneal nerve below the right knee.

chronic baroreflex dysfunction. Consistent with this, the weight of evidence suggests that the initial BP, HR, and MSNA responses to head-up tilt are normal in people who faint.[26,28,29]

However, there may be a subset of patients with subtle baroreflex dysfunction. Decreased sympathetic and vasoconstrictor responses to low-pressure baroreflexes have been reported.[27,44–46] Others have found decreased sympathetic,[47] vasoconstrictor,[48,49] and HR[50] responses to arterial baroreflexes. Reports of exaggerated low-pressure[51,52] and arterial baroreflex responses[53,54] are few. Some of these variations may be explained by recent studies demonstrating effects of gender and age on sympathetic baroreflex function.[55,56] Overall, evidence suggests that, although there may be a group of patients with syncope and impaired low-pressure baroreflexes, the vast

majority have arterial baroreflexes that are initially able to compensate for decreased venous return, at least during early head-up tilt. It has been argued that, although these arterial baroreflexes respond normally during initial orthostasis, they subsequently fail during the course of a vasovagal reaction.[57,58]

Progressive Early Hypotension

After a variable period of tilt, during which vasoconstriction compensates for decreased venous return and cardiac output, patients (and normal people) destined to develop tilt syncope enter into a phase the author termed "progressive early hypotension." This phase is marked by a gradual decrease in BP (a decrease in mean BP of about 20 mm Hg) during a variable period of up to

5 minutes. It is driven by a progressive decrease in cardiac output or both cardiac output and total peripheral resistance, despite a sustained increase in MSNA and HR.[30,39,59–61] There is little information from these studies as to whether the 2 different mechanisms relate to, for example, demographic variation between groups or subtle differences in baroreflex function (see earlier), but it seems that in most patients, a decrease in cardiac output is the dominant mechanism.[39,59,61]

The relationship between MSNA and total peripheral resistance during progressive early hypotension has been reported by Fu and colleagues[31] in a group of normal young adults (mean age 30 years, mainly women without a history of fainting, n = 25) during a short period (3 minutes) preceding tilt-induced syncope. Cardiac output decreased gradually in all subjects, associated with simultaneous vasodilatation in 16 of them, even though MSNA was maintained at increased levels, an example of a situation in which MSNA does not correlate with total peripheral resistance in the usual way.[32] The mechanism for vasodilatation here is uncertain and may relate to differential sympathetic activity (see earlier).[33] However, there are other possible mechanisms to consider. In young women, there is no clear relationship between MSNA and total peripheral resistance at rest, perhaps secondary to increased beta-2 adrenergic receptor–mediated vasodilatation.[62,63] It may be that "active vasodilatation" occurs to some degree in these subjects, but how important this is depends on how frequently it can be demonstrated in patients who regularly faint.[61] Other possible mechanisms that may explain general vasodilatation during increased MSNA include loss of nerve signal transduction (to the alpha adrenergic receptors),[64] increased nitric oxide activity,[65] and secretion of a circulating vasodilator.[66]

It is likely from the sequence of events described earlier, particularly in patients with vasoconstriction during presyncope, that stroke volume decreases secondary to decreased venous return.[67] Although 80% of the blood volume lies in venous capacitance vessels, very little is known about how they are controlled during VVS.[68] It is likely that the capacitance vessels (predominantly in the splanchnic bed) are most important with regard to venous return and cardiac output during orthostasis and progressive early hypotension. Studies from anesthetized animals have demonstrated that when splanchnic vasoconstriction occurs and arterial blood flow into capacitance vessels is decreased, the passive recoil of the veins overcomes the distending pressure and more blood is directed centrally to the heart.

There is another mechanism by which active venoconstriction of small veins (under sympathetic baroreflex control) may decrease venous compliance and further increase venous return. This active process is coordinated with arterial vasoconstriction by the baroreflexes but is considered less important than the passive mechanism.[68,69] Unfortunately, most studies in patients with syncope have measured venous compliance, whereas changes in capacitance (or the "unstressed volume") are more important.[70] It is clear that to understand the mechanisms involved in progressive early hypotension, one needs to know more about splanchnic venous capacitance and the sympathetic control thereof. For example, applying the above-mentioned mechanisms, how does the vasodilating group maintain cardiac output (assuming splanchnic vasodilatation is contributing) when venous return may be decreasing because of decreased passive emptying? Presumably active venoconstriction becomes more important here.

It has been demonstrated, using a radionucleotide technique, that patients with syncope have exaggerated splenic pooling of blood during exercise.[71] Stewart and colleagues[72] used impedance plethysmography during tilt to show that thoracic hypovolemia and splanchnic blood pooling were increased in patients with syncope (n = 34) compared with controls (n = 11). The same group demonstrated subsequently (by estimating blood flow from the impedance wave form) that splanchnic pooling in patients with syncope is associated with increased flow into these capacitance vessels,[73] suggesting that the mechanism here may be sympathetic-mediated splanchnic arterial vasodilatation, allowing more blood into the capacitance reservoir.

What about active venoconstriction? Unfortunately, the only data available come from peripheral veins, not from the splanchnic circulation. Venoconstriction does not occur in the limbs of normal subjects during tilt, and peripheral venous hemodynamics in patients with syncope are normal.[74,75] Furthermore, in patients with syncope, calf volume changes in the lower limbs during thigh cuff inflation bear no relationship to tilt tolerance and data on calf volume changes during tilt are controversial.[76,77] It may be that patients with syncope have abnormal control of venoconstriction in response to mental stress.[78] Peripheral venous pressure has not been measured systematically during progressive early hypotension and has not been demonstrated to increase before syncope.[79] Perhaps the strongest evidence for the importance of capacitance comes from the observation that during progressive early hypotension, syncope can be postponed by mechanisms known to increase venous return, for example, muscle tensing, leg crossing, and inflating an antigravity suit,[80,81] suggesting that venous pooling may decrease central venous pressure, stroke volume, and cardiac output during this part of the sequence.[82,83]

Terminal Vasodilatation

During the last 2 minutes before syncope, the next phase of the "vasovagal sequence" takes over, which the author calls "terminal vasodilatation." BP starts to decrease rapidly (usually, mean BP decreases a further 40 mm Hg during this time), associated with withdrawal of MSNA and slowing of HR.[26–29] The first MSNA studies reported bursts to disappear or decrease considerably, but later work found that total withdrawal may be unusual.[30,84] Burst width (and therefore burst size) increased in several patients during syncope (**Fig. 3**).[85] Therefore, depending on what modality is measured, it seems that in some patients MSNA is maintained or even increased when BP plummets, and once again, the normal sympathoconstrictor mechanism is disrupted. In most patients, however, there is at least partial MSNA withdrawal and terminal vasodilatation irrespective of the mechanism of hypotension during the previous phase. This finding means that for the group that has vasoconstriction during progressive early hypotension, the profile for total peripheral resistance becomes biphasic, whereas in the other group, vasodilatation is progressive throughout. There does not appear to be any relationship between the dominant hemodynamic process during presyncope (gradual vasodilatation or vasoconstriction) and the pattern of MSNA withdrawal later on.

HR decreases immediately before syncope, nearly always after the rapid decrease in BP and sympathetic withdrawal.[86] This condition is usually associated with hypotensive symptoms.[26–29] Slowing of the HR invariably results in decreased MSNA burst frequency because sympathetic bursts are gated to HR.[25] When the mean BP decreases to less than 60 mm Hg (at heart level) or the heart stops for more than 7 seconds, the cerebral ischemic anoxia reserve threshold is reached and consciousness is lost.[87] In practice, patients are usually tilted back to the horizontal before this occurs, resulting in almost immediate recovery of BP. In a related reflex condition, carotid sinus sensitivity, when cardiac output is decreased by extreme bradycardia during sinus massage, sympathetic withdrawal and vasodilatation further prolong recovery of BP (**Fig. 4**).[88] Therefore, even pacing patients in this situation does not normalize cardiac output, and BP continues to decrease because of the inherent latency of the sympathoconstrictor mechanism. The same interaction may apply when sympathetic withdrawal occurs with bradycardia during VVS. This condition is reflected in the rather disappointing results from permanent pacemaker insertion in most patients with VVS.[89]

Prolonged Postfaint Hypotension

An interesting observation from tilt studies is that not all patients recover their BP immediately on assuming the horizontal position. Some remain

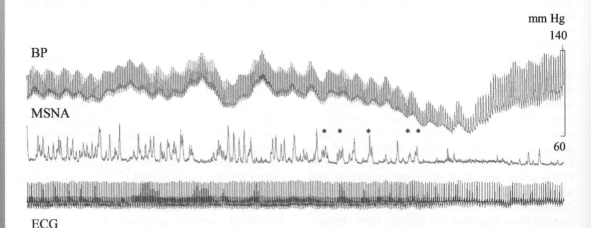

Fig. 3. A typical example of tilt-induced syncope (2-min tracings) showing changes in morphology of the MSNA bursts during terminal vasodilatation. In this patient, the burst amplitudes get smaller during the last minute before blood pressure nadir, but some of the bursts become broader (*asterisk*) because adjacent bursts fuse together. This condition becomes more noticeable as heart rate slows. Therefore, burst frequency also decreases as the heart rate slows.

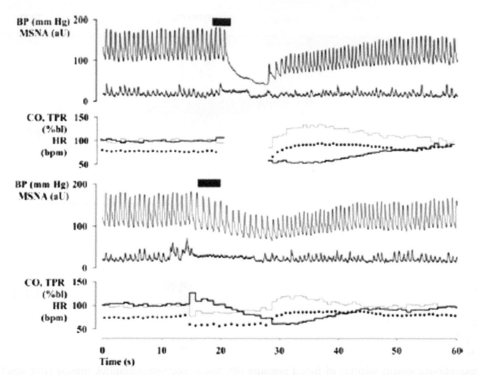

Fig. 4. Blood pressure (BP), muscle sympathetic nerve activity (MSNA), cardiac output (*gray line*, CO), heart rate (*dotted line*, HR), and total peripheral resistance (*black line*, TPR) during asystole induced by carotid sinus massage without (*top panel*) and with (*bottom panel*) demand pacing. Note that in both panels there is complete withdrawal of MSNA and major vasodilatation during asystole, which means that BP continues to decrease despite pacing. Time and duration of massage is denoted by thick black bars. (*From* Krediet CT, Jardine DL, Wieling W. Dissection of carotid sinus hypersensitivity: the timing of vagal and vasodepressor effects and the effect of body position. Clin Sci (Lond) 2011;121:389–96; with permission. © the Biochemical Society.)

pale, unwell, and hypotensive for up to 5 minutes, with vagal (usually gastrointestinal) symptoms.[90] The mechanism for this prolonged reaction has been demonstrated to be delayed recovery of stroke volume and cardiac output, not protracted vasodilatation and sympathetic withdrawal.[91] Therefore, excess vagal activity, possibly inhibiting cardiac contractility and cardiac output, may be a factor prolonging recovery in some patients.[92] Just how important this mechanism is immediately before syncope when cardiovagal activity becomes apparent is unknown.

RESPIRATION

For reasons that are unclear, respiration is stimulated before syncope, and this may indirectly exacerbate systemic hypotension and increase cerebrovascular resistance.[93] The increase in respiration (usually mediated by tidal volume) probably starts during progressive early hypotension, before hypotensive symptoms become apparent.[73,93] Although the vascular effects of hyperventilation may be relatively enhanced in

patients with recurrent syncope, it seems that the effect on cerebral vasoconstriction is relatively minor and that systemic BP is considered to be far more important for maintaining cerebral perfusion during presyncope,[94,95] which is discussed later.

CEREBRAL AUTOREGULATION

The sequence must take into account the relationship between systemic BP and cerebral blood flow, because the final common pathway of all proposed mechanisms for VVS is decreased cerebral perfusion.[96] Cerebral autoregulation can be thought of as "static," referring to the steady-state relationship between cerebral blood flow and systemic BP during pharmacologic challenge.[97] There is currently no evidence that static cerebral autoregulation operates at a higher set point in patients with recurrent VVS than in controls, thereby predisposing them to loss of consciousness at higher BP levels during tilt testing.[98]

With the advent of transcranial Doppler, "dynamic" cerebral autoregulation (defined as

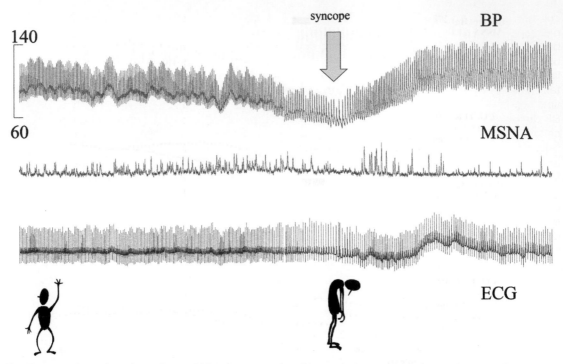

Fig. 5. Four-minute-length tracings of blood pressure (BP, finger plethysmography), muscle sympathetic nerve activity (MSNA), and electrocardiography (ECG) during tilt-induced syncope. For the first 2 minutes, decline in BP is slow and MSNA is maintained (progressive early hypotension). During the last 30 seconds before BP nadir, BP declines rapidly, MSNA withdraws, and HR slows (terminal vasodilatation).

cerebral blood flow responses to rapid changes in BP) has been studied. During progressive early hypotension, middle cerebral blood flow velocity and calculated cerebrovascular resistance decrease with systemic BP and cardiac output.[98–100] However, immediately before syncope, cerebral blood flow may become impaired by increased ventilation, causing

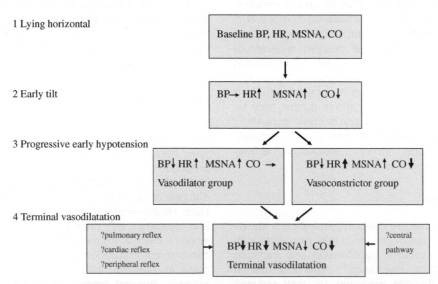

Fig. 6. The hemodynamic sequence involving blood pressure [BP], heart rate [HR], muscle nerve sympathetic activity [MSNA] and cardiac output [CO] before tilt-induced syncope. Phases 1 and 2 are similar for all patients but during progressive early hypotension, patients may undergo vasodilatation or vasoconstriction. During terminal vasodilatation, there is usually withdrawal of MSNA and both groups undergo vasodilatation despite a decrease in cardiac output. The trigger for this is uncertain.

collapse of intracerebral arterioles.[101] By this mechanism, the critical closing pressure of cerebral arterioles may increase, thereby decreasing blood flow distally. Therefore, the effects of ventilation on cerebral perfusion become very important during terminal vasodilatation. However, the time course and effects of ventilation on systemic BP during progressive early hypotension are less certain.

Dynamic cerebral autoregulation can also be analyzed using linear analysis, for example, transfer function. Indices derived from transfer function analyses (including gain, phase shift, and coherence) have been used to quantify the association between BP and cerebral blood flow waveforms during spontaneous BP fluctuations and tilt.[102] Coherence between BP and cerebral blood flow is less for low-frequency fluctuations (compared with high), suggesting that cerebral autoregulation is more active during these slow changes.[103] However, whether increased coherence between low-frequency fluctuations of BP during tilt-induced (mild) hypotension really means loss of cerebral autoregulation is uncertain.[104]

A further complicating factor is that cerebral autoregulation may be relatively less active during acute hypotension than hypertension.[105] Nonlinear analysis has found that during progressive early hypotension, respiratory oscillations may not only decrease cerebral autoregulation but also stimulate cardiovagal activity (possibly via pulmonary stretch receptors) and so be responsible for bradycardia and sympathetic withdrawal during terminal vasodilatation.[106] Therefore, increased respiration during presyncope may be the "missing link," providing a mechanism for the abrupt changes occurring immediately before syncope as an alternative to the neurocardiogenic reflex.

SUMMARY

There are inherent difficulties when trying to integrate different studies for the purposes of understanding the hemodynamic sequence before syncope (**Figs. 5** and **6**). The sequence the author outlines is as follows: most patients with recurrent VVS have normal baseline sympathohemodynamics and arterial baroreflex function. After an appropriate adjustment to orthostasis, patients subsequently experience a gradual decrease in BP for a few minutes. In some, this is secondary to decreased cardiac output, while in others it is secondary to simultaneously decreased cardiac output and vasodilatation. The author calls this phase *progressive early hypotension*. It is gradual in onset, relatively asymptomatic, and well

recognized by researchers despite several terminologies.[107,108] In patients who vasodilate, the relationship between MSNA and peripheral resistance during this phase is uncertain. After a variable time, all patients enter the next phase called *terminal vasodilatation*. The mechanism for this may be splanchnic blood pooling, thoracic hypovolemia, and increased ventilation, which in turn may decrease cerebral autoregulation and override the baroreflexes. The result is usually sympathetic withdrawal; a further, more rapid decrease in BP; and, finally, bradycardia. Syncope occurs secondary to decreased cerebral perfusion as a consequence of this. Recovery is immediate on restoration of venous return but may be prolonged in some patients by excess vagal activity, causing transiently impaired cardiac function.

ACKNOWLEDGMENTS

The author thanks all colleagues and coworkers who contributed to his research in Christchurch. This article is dedicated to the author's (recently departed) father Jim, a general surgeon, who, working before the advent of the CT scanner, was always wary of the signs of progressive central hypovolemia in patients with occult bleeding. He was a source of great encouragement.

REFERENCES

1. Colman N, Nahm K, van Dijk JG, et al. Diagnostic value of history taking in reflex syncope. Clin Auton Res 2004;14(Suppl I):I37–44.
2. Mosqueda-Garcia R, Furlan R, Tank J, et al. The elusive pathophysiology of neurally mediated syncope. Circulation 2000;102:2898–906.
3. Colman N, Nahm K, Ganzeboom KS, et al. Epidemiology of syncope. Clin Auton Res 2004; 14(Suppl I):I9–17.
4. Thijs RD, Wieling W, Kaufmann H, et al. Defining and classifying syncope. Clin Auton Res 2004; 14(Suppl I):I4–8.
5. Oberg B, White S. The role of vagal cardiac nerves and arterial baroreceptors in the circulatory adjustments to hemorrhage in the cat. Acta Physiol Scand 1970;80:395–403.
6. Ludbrook J, Ventura S. Roles of carotid baroreceptor and cardiac afferents in hemodynamic responses to acute central hypovolemia. Am J Physiol Heart Circ Physiol 1996;270:H1538–48.
7. Gauer OH, Henry JP. Negative [-Gz] acceleration in relation to arterial oxygen saturation, subendocardial hemorrhage and venous pressure in the forehead. Aerosp Med 1964;35:533–45.

8. Thoren P. The role of cardiac vagal C-fibres in cardiovascular control. Rev Physiol Biochem Pharmacol 1979;86:1–94.

9. Jarisch A, Zotterman Y. Depressor reflexes from the heart. Acta Physiol Scand 1948;16:31–51.

10. van Dijk JG. Fainting in animals. Clin Auton Res 2003;13:247–55.

11. Fitzpatrick AP, Banner N, Cheng A, et al. Vasovagal reactions may occur after orthotopic heart transplantation. J Am Coll Cardiol 1993;21:1132–7.

12. Scherrer U, Vissing S, Morgan BJ, et al. Vasovagal syncope after infusion of a vasodilator in a heart transplant recipient. N Engl J Med 1990;322:602–4.

13. Kinsella SM, Tuckey JP. Perioperative bradycardia and asystole: relationship to vasovagal syncope and the Bezold-Jariisch reflex. Br J Anaesth 2001;86:859–68.

14. Shalev Y, Rami G, Tchou PJ, et al. Echocardiographic demonstration of decreased left ventricular dimensions and vigorous myocardial contraction during syncope induced by head-up tilt. J Am Coll Cardiol 1991;18:746–51.

15. Yamanouchi Y, Jaalouk S, Shehadeh AA, et al. Changes in left ventricular volume during head-up tilt in patients with vasovagal syncope: an echocardiographic study. Am Heart J 1996;131:73–80.

16. Novak V, Honos G, Schondorf R. Is the heart empty at syncope? J Auton Nerv Syst 1996;60:83–92.

17. Hainsworth R. Syncope: what is the trigger? Heart 2003;89:123–4.

18. Wesseling KH. Continuous non-invasive recording of arterial pressure. Homeostasis 1995;36:50–66.

19. Imholz BP, Wieling W, van Montfrans G, et al. Fifteen years experience with finger pressure monitoring; assessment of the technology. Cardiovasc Res 1998;38:605–16.

20. Jellema WT, Wesseling KH, Groeneveld AB, et al. Continuous cardiac output in septic shock by simulating a model of the aortic impedance. Anesthesiology 1999;90:1317–28.

21. Murray RH, Thompson LJ, Bowers JA, et al. Hemodynamic effects of graded hypovolemia and vasodepressor syncope induced by lower body negative pressure. Am Heart J 1968;76:799–811.

22. Stevens PM. Cardiovascular dynamics during orthostasis and the influence of intravascular instrumentation. Am J Cardiol 1966;17:211–8.

23. Bergenwald L, Freyschuss U, Sjostrand T. The mechanism of orthostatic and hemorrhagic fainting. Scand J Clin Lab Invest 1977;37:209–16.

24. Glick G, Yu P. Hemodynamic changes during spontaneous vasovagal reactions. Am J Med 1963;34:42–51.

25. Valbo AB, Haqbath K, Wallin DQ. Microneurography: how the technique developed and its role in the investigation of the sympathetic nervous system. J Appl Physiol 2004;96:1262–9.

26. Morillo CA, Eckberg DL, Ellenbogen KA, et al. Vagal and sympathetic mechanisms in patients with orthostatic vasovagal syncope. Circulation 1997;96:2509–13.

27. Mosqueda-Garcia R, Furlan R, Fernandez-Violante R, et al. Sympathetic and baroreceptor reflex function in neurally mediated syncope evoked by tilt. J Clin Invest 1997;99:2736–44.

28. Jardine DL, Ikram H, Frampton CM, et al. The autonomic control of vasovagal syncope. Am J Physiol Heart Circ Physiol 1998;274:H2110–5.

29. Kamiya A, Hayano J, Kawada T, et al. Low-frequency oscillation of sympathetic nerve activity decreases during development of tilt-induced syncope preceding sympathetic withdrawal and bradycardia. Am J Physiol Heart Circ Physiol 2005;289:H1758–69.

30. Cooke WH, Rickards CA, Ryan KL, et al. Muscle sympathetic activity during intense lower body negative pressure to presyncope in humans. J Physiol 2009;587:4987–99.

31. Fu QI, Verheyden B, Wieling W, et al. Cardiac output and sympathetic vasoconstrictor responses during upright tilt to presyncope in healthy humans. J Physiol 2012;590:1839–48.

32. Fu Q, Shook RP, Okazaki K, et al. Vasomotor sympathetic neural control is maintained during sustained upright posture in humans. J Physiol 2006;577:679–87.

33. Morrison SF. Differential control of sympathetic flow. Am J Physiol Regul Integr Comp Physiol 2001;281:R683–98.

34. Rowell LB, Detry J, Blackmon JR, et al. Importance of the splanchnic vascular bed in human blood pressure regulation. J Appl Physiol 1972;332:213–20.

35. Rowell LB. Reflex control of regional circulations in humans. J Auton Nerv Syst 1984;11:101–14.

36. Deharo J, Jego C, Lanteaume A, et al. An implatable loop recorder study of highly symptomatic vasovagal patients. J Am Coll Cardiol 2006;47:587–93.

37. Moya A, Brignole M, Menozzi C, et al. Mechanism of syncope in patients with isolated syncope and in patients with tilt-positive syncope. Circulation 2001;104:1261–7.

38. Vadaadi G, Corcoran SJ, Esler M. Management strategies for recurrent vasovagal syncope. Intern Med J 2010;40:554–60.

39. Jardine DL, Melton IC, Crozier IG, et al. Decrease in cardiac output and sympathetic activity during vasovagal syncope. Am J Physiol Heart Circ Physiol 2001;282:H1004–9.

40. Parati G, Parati G, Di Rienzo M, et al. How to measure baroreflex sensitivity: from the cardiovascular laboratory to daily life. J Hypertens 2000;18:7–19.

41. van Lieshout JJ, Wieling W, Karemaker JM. Neural circulatory control in vasovagal syncope. Pacing Clin Electrophysiol 1997;20:753–63.
42. Taylor JA, Halliwill JR, Brown TE, et al. Non-hypotensive hypovolaemia reduces ascending aortic dimensions in humans. J Physiol 1995;483:289–98.
43. Floras JS, Butler GC, Ando S, et al. Differential sympathetic nerve and heart rate spectral effects of non-hypotensive lower body negative pressure. Am J Physiol Regul Integr Comp Physiol 2001; 281:R468–75.
44. Thompson HL, Wright K, Frenneaux M. Baroreflex sensitivity in patients with vasovagal syncope. Circulation 1997;95:395–400.
45. Wasmund SL, Smith ML, Takata TS, et al. Sympathoexcitation is attenuated during low level lower body negative pressure in subjects who develop pre-syncope. Clin Auton Res 2003;13:208–13.
46. Wijeysundera DN, Butler GC, Ando S, et al. Attenuated cardiac baroreflex in men with presyncope evoked by lower body negative pressure. Clin Sci 2001;100:303–9.
47. Bechir M, Binggeli C, Corti FR, et al. Dysfunctional baroreflex regulation of sympathetic nerve activity in patients with vasovagal syncope. Circulation 2003;107:1620–5.
48. Brown CM, Hainsworth R. Forearm vascular responses during orthostasis in control subjects and patients with posturally related syncope. Clin Auton Res 2000;10:57–61.
49. Sneddon JF, Counihan PJ, Bashir Y, et al. Impaired immediate vasoconstrictor responses in patients with recurrent neurally mediated syncope. Am J Cardiol 1993;71:72–6.
50. Wahbha MM, Morley CA, Al-Sharma YM, et al. Cardiovascular reflex responses in patients with unexplained syncope. Clin Sci 1989;77:547–53.
51. Cooke WH, Convertino VA. Association between vasovagal hypotension and low sympathetic neural activity during presyncope. Clin Auton Res 2002; 12:483–6.
52. Sneddon JF, Bashir Y, Murgatroyd FD, et al. Do patients with neurally mediated syncope have augmented vagal tone? Am J Cardiol 1993;72: 1314–5.
53. Adler PS, France C, Ditto B. Baroreflex sensitivity at rest and during stress in individuals with a history of vasovagal syncope. J Psychosom Res 1991; 35:591–7.
54. Pitzalis M, Parati G, Massari F, et al. Enhanced reflex response to baroreceptor deactivation in subjects with tilt-induced syncope. J Am Coll Cardiol 2003;41:1167–73.
55. Hart EC, Joyner MJ, Wallin BG, et al. Sex, ageing and resting blood pressure: gaining insights from the integrated balance of neural and haemodynamic factors. J Physiol 2012;590:2069–79.
56. Shaw BH, Protheroe CL. Sex, drugs and blood pressure control: the impact of age and gender on sympathetic regulation of arterial pressure. J Physiol 2012;590:2841–3.
57. Ogoh S, Volianitis S, Raven PB, et al. Carotid baroreflex function ceases during vasovagal syncope. Clin Auton Res 2004;14:30–3.
58. Samniah N, Sakaguchi S, Ermis C, et al. Transient modification of baroreceptor response during tilt-induced vasovagal syncope. Europace 2004;6: 48–54.
59. Verheyden B, Liu J, van Dijk N, et al. Steep fall in cardiac output is main determinant of hypotension during drug-free and nitroglycerine-induced orthostatic vasovagal syncope. Heart Rhythm 2008;5: 1695–701.
60. Thomas KN, Galvin SD, Williams MJ, et al. Identical pattern of cerebral hypoperfusion during different types of syncope. J Hum Hypertens 2010;24: 458–66.
61. Fuca G, Dinelli M, Suzzani P, et al. The venous system is the main determinant of hypotension in patients with vasovagal syncope. Europace 2006; 8:839–45.
62. Hart EC, Charkoudian N, Wallin BG, et al. Sex differences in sympathetic neural-hemodynamic balance: implications for human blood pressure regulation. Hypertension 2009;53:571–6.
63. Hart EC, Charkoudian N, Wallin BG, et al. Sex and ageing differences in resting arterial pressure regulation: the role of the beta-adrenergic redceptors. J Physiol 2011;589:5285–97.
64. Charcoudian N, Joyner MJ, Sokolnicki LA, et al. Vascular adrenergic responsiveness is inversely related to tonic activity of sympathetic vasoconstrictor nerves in humans. J Physiol 2006;572: 821–7.
65. Dietz NM, Halliwill JR, Spielmann JM, et al. Sympathetic withdrawal and forearm vasodilation during vasovagal syncope in humans. J Appl Physiol 1997;82:1785–93.
66. Goldstein DS, Holmes C, Frank SM, et al. Sympathoadrenal imbalance before neurocardiogenic syncope. Am J Cardiol 2003;91:53–8.
67. Guyton AC, Lindsey AW, Aberrnathy B, et al. Venous return at various atrial pressures and the normal venous return curve. Am J Physiol 1957; 189:609–15.
68. Rothe CF. Reflex control of veins and vascular capacitance. Physiol Rev 1983;63:1281–342.
69. Rothe CF. Physiology of venous return: an unappreciated boost to the heart. Arch Intern Med 1986; 146:977–82.
70. Halliwill JR, Minson CT, Joyner MJ. Measurement of limb venous compliance in humans: technical considerations and physiological findings. J Appl Physiol 1999;87:1555–63.

71. Thomson HL, Atherton JJ, Khafagi FA, et al. Failure of reflex venoconstriction during exercise in patients with vasovagal syncope. Circulation 1996;93:953–9.

72. Stewart JM, Mcloed KJ, Sanyal S, et al. Relation of postural vasovagal syncope to splanchnic hypervolemia in adolescents. Circulation 2004;110:2575–81.

73. Taneja I, Medow MS, Glover JL, et al. Increased vasoconstriction predisposes to hyperpnea and postural faint. Am J Physiol Heart Circ Physiol 2008;295:H372–81.

74. Stewart JM, Weldon A. Contrasting neurovascular findings in clinical orthostatic intolerance and neurocardiogenic syncope. Clin Sci 2003;104:329–40.

75. Stewart JM, Lavin J, Weldon A. Orthostasis fails to produce active limb venoconstriction in adolescents. J Appl Physiol 2001;91:1723–9.

76. Bellard E, Fortrat J, Dupuis J, et al. Haemodynamic response to peripheral venous congestion in patients with unexplained recurrent syncope. Clin Sci 2003;105:331–7.

77. Hargreaves AD, Muir AL. Lack of variation in venous tone potentiates vasovagal syncope. Br Heart J 1992;67:486–90.

78. Manyari DE, Rose S, Tyberg JV, et al. Abnormal reflex function in patients with neuromediated syncope. J Am Coll Cardiol 1996;27:1370–735.

79. Epstein SE, Stampfer M, Beiser GD. Role of capacitance vessels in vasovagal syncope. Circulation 1968;37:524–33.

80. Krediet CT, van Dijk N, Linzer M, et al. Management of vasovagal syncope: controlling or aborting faints by leg crossing and muscle tensing. Circulation 2002;106:1684–9.

81. Weissler AM, Warren JV, Estes E, et al. Vasodepressor syncope: factors influencing cardiac output. Circulation 1957;15:875–82.

82. van Dijk N, de Bruin IG, Gisolf J, et al. Hemodynamic effects of leg crossing and skeletal muscle tensing during free standing in patients with vasovagal syncope. J Appl Physiol 2005;98:584–90.

83. van Lieshout JJ, Pott F, Madsen PL, et al. Muscle tensing during standing: effects on cerebral tissue oxygenation and cerebral artery blood velocity. Stroke 2001;32:1546–51.

84. Vadaadi G, Esler MD, Dawood T, et al. Persistence of muscle sympathetic nerve activity during vasovagal syncope. Eur Heart J 2010;31:2027–33.

85. Iwase S, Mano T, Kamiya A, et al. Syncopal attack alters the burst properties of muscle sympathetic nerve activity in humans. Auton Neurosci 2002;95:141–5.

86. Schroeder C, Tank J, Heusser K, et al. Physiological phenomenology of neurally mediated syncope with management of complications. PLoS One 2011;6:1–8.

87. Wieling W, Thijs RD, van Dijk N, et al. Symptoms and signs of syncope: a review of the link between physiology and clinical clues. Brain 2009;132:2630–42.

88. Krediet CT, Jardine DL, Wieling W. Dissection of carotid sinus hypersensitivity: the timing of vagal and vasodepressor effects and the effect of body position. Clin Sci 2011;121:389–96.

89. Brignole M, Menozzi C, Moya A, et al. Pacemaker therapy in patients with neurally mediated syncope and documented asystole: third International Study on Syncope of Uncertain Etiology [ISSUE 3]: a randomised trial. Circulation 2012;125:2566–71.

90. Wieling W, Rozenberg J, Go-Schön IK, et al. Hemodynamic mechanisms underlying prolonged postfaint hypotension. Clin Auton Res 2011;21:405–13.

91. Rozenberg J, Wieling W, Schon IK, et al. MSNA during prolonged post-faint hypotension. Clin Auton Res 2012;22:167–73.

92. Casadei B. Vagal control of myocardial contractility in humans. Exp Physiol 2001;86:817–23.

93. Lagi A, Cencetti S, Corsoni V, et al. Cerebral vasoconstriction in vasovagal syncope: any link with symptoms? Circulation 2001;104:2694–8.

94. Norcliffe-Kaufmann L, Kaufmann H, Hainsworth R. Enhanced vascular responses to hypocapnia in neurally mediated syncope. Ann Neurol 2008;63:288–94.

95. Levine BD, Giller CA, Lane LD, et al. Cerebral versus systemic hemodynamics during graded orthostatic stress in humans. Circulation 1994;90:298–306.

96. Ainslie PN, Smith KJ. Integrated human physiology: breathing, blood pressure and blood flow to the brain. J Physiol 2011;589:2917.

97. Lassen NA. Cerebral blood flow and oxygen consumption in man. Physiol Rev 1959;39:183–238.

98. Carey BJ, Manktelow BN, Panerai RB, et al. Cerebral autoregulatory responses to head-up tilt in normal subjects and patients with recurrent vasovagal syncope. Circulation 2001;104:898–902.

99. Murrell C, Cotter JD, George K, et al. Influence of age on syncope following prolonged exercise: differential responses but similar orthostatic tolerance. J Physiol 2009;587:5959–69.

100. Schondorf R, Benoit J, Wein T. Cerebrovascular and cardiovascular measurements during neurally mediatedy syncope induced by head-up tilt. Stroke 1997;28:1564–8.

101. Carey BJ, Eames PJ, Panerai RB, et al. Carbon dioxide, critical closing pressure and cerebral haemodynamics prior to vasovagal syncope in humans. Clin Sci 2001;101:351–8.

102. van Beek AH, Classen JA, Rikkert MG, et al. Cerebral autoregulation: an overview of current concepts and methodology with special focus on

the elderly. J Cereb Blood Flow Metab 2008;28: 1071–85.

103. Zhang R, Zuckerman JH, Levine BD. Deterioration of cerebral autoregulation during orthostatic stress: insights from the frequency domain. J Appl Physiol 1998;85:1113–22.

104. Romero SA, Moralez G, Rickards CA, et al. Control of cerebral blood velocity with furosemide-induced hypovolemia and upright tilt. J Appl Physiol 2011; 110:492–8.

105. Tzeng Y, Willie CK, Atkinson G, et al. Cerebrovascular regulation during transient hypotension and hypertension in humans. Hypertension 2010;56: 268–73.

106. Ocon AJ, Medow MS, Taneja I, et al. Respiration drives phase synchronization between blood pressure and RR interval following loss of cardiovagal baroreflex during vasovagal syncope. Am J Physiol Heart Circ Physiol 2011;300:H527–40.

107. Joyner MJ. Orthostatic stress, haemorrhage and a bankrupt cardiovascular system. J Physiol 2009;587:5015–6.

108. Hainsworth R. Pathophysiology of syncope. Clin Auton Res 2004;14(Suppl I):I18–24.

Confounders of Vasovagal Syncope: Orthostatic Hypotension

Victor C. Nwazue, MD[a,b], Satish R. Raj, MD, MSCI[a,b],*

KEYWORDS

- Syncope • Vasovagal syncope • Orthostatic hypotension • Autonomic dysfunction
- Blood pressure

KEY POINTS

- Most patients who present with syncope have vasovagal (reflex) syncope, but neurogenic orthostatic hypotension can also cause syncope, especially in older patients.
- Patients with neurogenic orthostatic hypotension have a fall in blood pressure greater than or equal to 20/10 mm Hg within 3 minutes of assumption of an upright posture.
- Neurogenic orthostatic hypotension can often be differentiated from vasovagal syncope by its differing hemodynamic patterns during tilt table test and differing clinical characteristics.
- Treatment of orthostatic hypotension focuses on improving symptoms through careful attention to hydration; bolus ingestion of water (osmopressor response); and the judicious use of short-acting pressor agents.
- A significant proportion of patients with orthostatic hypotension can also have supine hypertension, which may necessitate the use of short-acting pressor agents overnight.

NOT ALL SYNCOPE IS VASOVAGAL SYNCOPE, EVEN WITH A NORMAL HEART

Cardiologists are trained to assess syncope patients for life-threatening causes. This usually involves a detailed evaluation to exclude valvular heart diseases, myocardial diseases, and cardiac arrhythmia. After these potentially lethal causes of syncope have been excluded, most cases are ascribed to vasovagal syncope (VVS). Cardiologists working in a syncope clinic or in a tilt table laboratory quickly realize that there are other causes for

syncope and presyncope, including neurogenic orthostatic hypotension (nOH) and postural tachycardia syndrome. This article highlights some contrasting clinical characteristics between nOH and VVS (**Table 1**), and then reviews the clinical evaluation and management of nOH. The clinical characteristics of postural tachycardia syndrome are reviewed elsewhere in this issue.

A striking difference between nOH and VVS is the different hemodynamic patterns during tilt table tests. These disorders each can have a distinct hemodynamic pattern during tilt table testing.

Research Funding: Supported in part by NIH grants R01 HL102387, P01 HL56693, and UL1 TR000445 (Clinical and Translational Science Award).

Conflicts of Interest: None.

[a] Division of Clinical Pharmacology, Department of Medicine, Autonomic Dysfunction Center, Vanderbilt University School of Medicine, AA3228 Medical Center North, 1161 21st Avenue South, Nashville, TN 37232–2195, USA; [b] Division of Clinical Pharmacology, Department of Pharmacology, Autonomic Dysfunction Center, Vanderbilt University School of Medicine, AA3228 Medical Center North, 1161 21st Avenue South, Nashville, TN 37232–2195, USA

* Corresponding author. Division of Clinical Pharmacology, Departments of Medicine and Pharmacology, Autonomic Dysfunction Center, Vanderbilt University School of Medicine, AA3228 Medical Center North, 1161 21st Avenue South, Nashville, TN 37232–2195.

E-mail address: satish.raj@vanderbilt.edu

Table 1
Clinical comparison of vasovagal syncope and neurogenic orthostatic hypotension

Features	Vasovagal Syncope	Neurogenic Orthostatic Hypotension
Typical age	Any age; first episode usually in second or third decade	>50 y
Gender (% female)	60%	40%
Symptoms with body position change	After prolonged sitting or standing	Immediately with sitting or standing
Syncope	+++	++
Presyncope	+	+++
Orthostatic Hypotension	+/- (usually only at time of faint)	+++++
Hemodynamic pattern with head-up tilt	Sudden drop in BP and HR	Early and progressive decline in BP

Abbreviations: BP, blood pressure; HR, heart rate.

During head-up tilt patients with VVS often hold a steady blood pressure (BP) for several minutes (often >10 minutes) after head-up tilt, before they develop symptoms and drop their BP rapidly (**Fig. 1**A). Patients with nOH are not able to maintain BP with head-up tilt. Their BP starts to fall immediately and orthostatic hypotension usually develops within 2 to 3 minutes of tilt (see **Fig. 1**B).

HEMODYNAMIC PHYSIOLOGY OF STANDING: HEALTHY AND ORTHOSTATIC HYPOTENSION

With the assumption of an upright posture, there is a downward shift of approximately 500 mL of blood to the dependent areas (mainly abdomen

and legs). This gravitational shift in blood results in decreased venous return, decreased cardiac output, and eventually decreased BP (**Fig. 2**A).[1] This "unloads" the baroreceptors, and triggers a reflex sympathetic activation with a resultant increase in heart rate (HR) and systemic vasoconstriction (countering the initial decline in BP). In a healthy individual, the net effect of assumption of upright posture is an increase in HR of 10 to 20 bpm, a minimal change in systolic BP, and an approximately 5 mm Hg increase in diastolic BP.

In patients with nOH (see **Fig. 2**B), the efferent limb of the baroreflex cannot be adequately engaged. This can result in a lack of sympathetically

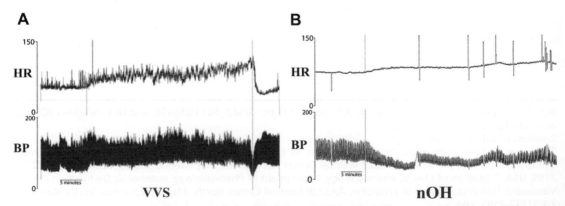

Fig. 1. Head-up tilt test traces from a patient with VVS and nOH. (*A*) With VVS, the heart rate (HR) and BP increase a little bit at the onset of tilt, and they are maintained for more than 25 minutes before a sudden precipitous drop in BP before the table is returned to the supine position. (*B*) With nOH, the BP falls almost immediately when the table is tilted up with only minimal changes in HR. (*From* Raj SR, Sheldon RS. Head-up tilt-table test. In: Saksena S, Camm AJ, editors. Electrophysiological disorders of the heart. 2nd edition. New York: Saunders; 2012. p. 73–6–73–8; with permission.)

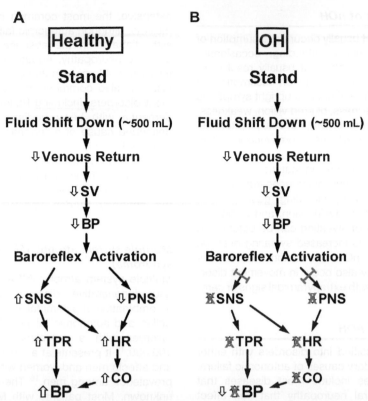

Fig. 2. Physiology of standing: healthy and orthostatic hypotension. (*A*) With standing, there is a downward shift of approximately 500 mL of blood, which results in decreased venous return, decreased stroke volume (SV), and eventually decreased BP. This "unloads" the baroreceptors, and triggers reflex sympathetic nervous system (SNS) activation with an increase in HR and systemic vasoconstriction (countering the initial decline in BP). In a healthy individual, the net effect of assumption of upright posture is an increase in HR of 10 to 20 bpm, a minimal change in systolic BP, and an approximately 5 mm Hg increase in diastolic BP. (*B*) In patients with OH, the SNS and parasympathetic nervous system (PNS) cannot be adequately engaged, so the counterregulation is absent, and a drop in BP occurs. CO, cardiac output; TPR, total peripheral resistance.

mediated vasoconstriction (and increase in vascular resistance) and a fixed HR, instead of the expected increased HR. Together, this physiology results in a lack of counterregulation and a drop in BP. If the cerebral perfusion pressure falls below a critical threshold (as can happen with systemic hypotension), then adequate cerebral blood flow is not maintained (despite cerebral autoregulation) and syncope or presyncope result.

NEUROGENIC ORTHOSTATIC HYPOTENSION

nOH is defined as a sustained decrease in systolic BP greater than or equal to 20 mm Hg or diastolic BP greater than or equal to 10 mm Hg within 3 minutes of the assumption of an upright posture,[2] although in almost all cases these diagnostic thresholds are met within 2 minutes.[3,4] More recent guidelines for patients with severe supine hypertension raise the threshold to a reduction in systolic BP greater than or equal to 30 mm Hg.[2]

"Delayed orthostatic hypotension" has also been described with orthostatic symptoms occurring after 3 minutes, and a slow gradual drop in BP that crosses the threshold BP drop after 3 minutes of upright posture.[2,5] Delayed nOH may represent a mild form of sympathetic nervous system failure.

The National Institutes of Health–funded longitudinal Framingham Heart study in the United States found that nOH accounted for 9.4% of all-cause syncope in their cohort.[6] A European study reported that up to 24% of syncope-associated complaints were associated with nOH during emergency room visits.[7]

nOH is more prevalent with increasing age, with an estimated prevalence rate of 18% in patients greater than or equal to 65 years of age,[8] and also represents a common cause of hospitalization among this age group.[9] Recent studies have found that the presence of nOH is a strong predictor of future cardiovascular events.[10]

Clinical Features of nOH

Symptoms of nOH usually occur on assumption of upright posture (usually standing, occasionally even while seated) and most usually resolve (or improve greatly) very rapidly on resumption of a recumbent posture. Common upright symptoms include lightheadedness, blurred vision, weakness, fatigue, cognitive impairment, nausea, palpitations, tremulousness, headache, presyncope, and syncope.[2] These symptoms are often incapacitating. In addition to the orthostatic symptoms, patients can often have other noncardiovascular autonomic symptoms, including gastroparesis, constipation, bladder dysfunction, and anhidrosis (although the loss of sweating can be patchy and may be reported as increased sweating over the face and chest). nOH and autonomic nervous system failure may also occur in movement disorders that present with extrapyramidal signs or cerebellar ataxia.

Classification of nOH

nOH can be classified into disorders with either primary or secondary causes of autonomic failure. Secondary causes include most diseases that cause a peripheral neuropathy that can affect the peripheral small fibers (including the autonomic nerves) (**Box 1**). Although this list is

---

Box 1
Causes of nOH

Primary autonomic failure

- Multiple system atrophy (Shy-Drager syndrome)
- Pure autonomic failure (Bradbury-Eggleston syndrome)
- Dementia with Lewy bodies

Secondary autonomic failure

- Diabetes mellitus
- Parkinson disease
- Amyloid
- Autoimmune autonomic ganglionopathy
- Guillain-Barré syndrome
- Familial dysautonomia (Riley-Day syndrome)
- Hereditary sensory autonomic neuropathy
- Vitamin deficiency (e.g. vitamin B_{12})
- Toxic neuropathy
- Drug-induced neuropathy
- Infectious neuropathy

---

extensive, the most common cause is diabetes mellitus, although autonomic failure is uncommon with diabetes in the absence of a glove and stocking neuropathy. Another cause of a potentially reversible neuropathy is amyloid. Autonomic failure is also commonly associated with movement disorders, including Parkinson disease and dementia with Lewy bodies. A more recently described cause of autonomic failure is autoimmune autonomic ganglionopathy. In this disorder, an autoantibody targeting the autonomic ganglia causes loss of function and autonomic failure.[11] In some cases, treatments targeted at reducing the antibody burden improve or resolve the nOH.[12–14]

Multiple system atrophy (Shy-Drager syndrome)

Multiple system atrophy (MSA) is a progressive, neurodegenerative disease characterized by a combination of pyramidal, extrapyramidal, cerebellar, and autonomic failure. MSA is a sporadic disorder with a prevalence of 4 to 5 per 100,000.[15] It presents at a mean age of 54 years, and affects men and women with a slightly higher prevalence among men.[16] The cause of MSA is unknown. Most patients with MSA present with autonomic complaints (e.g., bladder dysfunction, erectile dysfunction, constipation, or nOH), but develop motor symptoms within 2 years.[17] Most patients with MSA (approximately 80%) have Parkinson-like motor features, with a smaller number having predominantly cerebellar motor symptoms.[18] Patients with MSA can often be differentiated from patients with Parkinson disease by their poor response to therapy with levodopa. MSA presents with a very poor prognosis with a median survival of only 7 to 9 years[19] from the point of diagnosis, and a progressively debilitating course until death.[20]

MSA can be grouped into three major diagnostic groups[21]: (1) definite MSA, for patients with autopsy demonstration of typical histopathologic features; (2) probable MSA, for patients with multiple features of autonomic failure in addition to extrapyramidal or ataxic motor symptoms; and (3) possible MSA, for patients with less classical clinical findings. Many patients do not receive the correct diagnosis of MSA while alive because of the difficulty in differentiating MSA from other disorders (e.g., Parkinson disease, or other rare movement disorders). The defining neuropathologic findings of MSA consist of degeneration of striatonigral and olivopontocerebellar structures accompanied by profuse distinctive glial cytoplasmic inclusions formed by fibrillized α-synuclein proteins.[21–23] Clinically, one can only make a diagnosis of possible MSA or probable MSA. **Table 2** summarizes some clinical features of MSA (central autonomic failure).

Differentiating MSA from Parkinson disease

Most patients with MSA have parkinsonian features, which can clinically mimic Parkinson disease. These include a resting tremor (more often bilateral in MSA than Parkinson disease); bradykinesia; rigidity; and postural instability. Both groups of patients can develop autonomic failure and orthostatic hypotension, although this typically occurs earlier in the course of MSA and later in the course of Parkinson disease.

One important distinguishing clinical feature is that patients with Parkinson disease usually experience a dramatic reduction in muscle stiffness with L-dopa replacement therapy (e.g., Sinemet), whereas patients with MSA often have a poor clinical response. The diagnosis often becomes clearer over time, because patients with MSA experience a more rapid clinical deterioration than patients with Parkinson disease.

Although Parkinson disease and dementia with Lewy bodies have central nervous system features, the autonomic failure in Parkinson disease is caused by a peripheral autonomic neuropathy and behaves like pure autonomic failure (see **Table 2**).[24] These disorders can manifest evidence of cardiac sympathetic nerve

degeneration,[25] similar to that shown in **Fig. 3** using *m*-iodobenzylguanidine scans of the heart.

Pure autonomic failure (idiopathic orthostatic hypotension, Bradbury-Eggleston syndrome)

Pure autonomic failure was first described by Bradbury and Eggleston in 1925.[26] They described patients with orthostatic hypotension who had an unchanging HR, supine hypertension, reduced sweating, impotence, nocturia, constipation, and anemia. These patients had failure of the sympathetic and parasympathetic limbs of the autonomic nervous system, and "denervation hypersensitivity" in response to pharmacologic agonists. Compression garments helped these patients, presumably by preventing the pooling of blood in the lower body.

Pure autonomic failure is a disease process primarily involving the peripheral autonomic nerves. Autonomic neurons develop aggregates of a housekeeping protein called α-synuclein in the cytoplasm, known as Lewy bodies. These Lewy bodies damage the neurons. Lewy bodies are also seen in Parkinson disease and dementia with Lewy bodies. In contrast, patients with MSA have inclusions in glial cells and not neurons.

The clinical characteristics of pure autonomic failure (compared with MSA) are shown in **Table 2**. Patients with pure autonomic failure tend to develop their symptoms in their seventh decade

Table 2 Central versus peripheral autonomic failure		
	Central Autonomic Failure	**Peripheral Autonomic Failure**
Pathologic Lesions		
Lesion	Preganglionic	Postganglionic
Clinical features		
Orthostatic hypotension	+++++	+++++
Supine hypertension	~50%	~50%
Falls	+++	++
Olfactory function	Normal	Decreased
Nocturia	+++	+++
Laboratory testing		
Supine plasma NE	Normal	Low
Standing plasma NE	Low	Low
Orthostatic plasma NE	Minimal or no increase	Minimal or no increase
Cardiac SNS innervation (^{123}I-MIBG scan)	Normal	Decreased
Quantitative sudomotor axonal reflex testing	Can be normal	Abnormal at multiple sites
Thermoregulatory sweat test	Abnormal	Abnormal

Abbreviations: MIBG, *m*-iodobenzylguanidine; NE, norepinephrine; SNS, sympathetic nervous system.

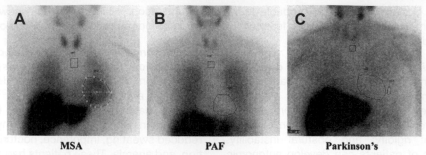

MSA   **PAF**   **Parkinson's**

Fig. 3. Cardiac sympathetic nerve integrity. Cardiac sympathetic nerve integrity can be assessed with *m*-iodoben-zylguanidine (MIBG) scans with a chest view at 4 hours postinjection. MIBG is taken up by intact presynaptic norepinephrine transporters on postganglionic sympathetic neurons, and is not present in the setting of significant postganglionic sympathetic neuropathy. In MSA (*A*), the lesions are central and preganglionic. Because there is not postganglionic involvement, the heart takes up MIBG avidly. In contrast, patients with pure autonomic failure (PAF) (*B*) have a significant postganglionic sympathetic neuropathy, and the heart cannot be seen because it cannot take up MIBG. (*C*) Scan of a patient with Parkinson disease. Although the motor features of Parkinson disease are caused by central nervous system lesions, the autonomic failure is caused by a peripheral postganglionic sympathetic neuropathy, with poor cardiac uptake of MIBG.

or later, and have a fairly good prognosis with a slow progression. As a result of the peripheral autonomic nerve damage, patients with pure autonomic failure have a significantly lower supine level of plasma norepinephrine than do healthy age-matched control subjects.[27]

Evaluation of nOH

A good history and physical examination remains the single most valuable diagnostic resource. Non-neurologic causes of orthostatic hypotension, such as dehydration, acute blood loss, and deleterious medications, should be identified because these can be reversed. nOH can also be mimicked by disorders with decreased cardiac output, such as cardiomyopathy, constrictive pericarditis, and aortic stenosis.[28] The critical element of making a diagnosis of nOH involves obtaining orthostatic vital signs (BP and HR) in response to upright posture for at least 3 minutes, and ideally for 5 minutes.[3] A diagnosis of nOH cannot be made in the absence of orthostatic vital signs. **Box 2** lists several orthostatic and nonorthostatic symptoms commonly seen in patients with nOH. Initial blood tests should commonly include a complete blood count (to exclude severe anemia); electrolytes; serum vitamin B_{12} levels; and serum and urine immunoelectrophoresis (to exclude monoclonal proteins that might cause amyloid neuropathy).[28]

Autonomic function testing in nOH
Formal autonomic function testing can be done in special centers and is integral to the diagnosis of autonomic failure. Testing assesses the parasympathetic nervous system and the sympathetic nervous system. Cardiovagal function can be assessed with a quantitative assessment of HR

excursion with respiration (sinus arrhythmia), and the HR response to a Valsalva maneuver.[29] The sympathetic cholinergic nervous system can be assessed with sweat tests (the quantitative

Box 2
Common symptoms with orthostatic hypotension

Orthostatic symptoms (worse with upright posture)
- Lightheadedness
- Presyncope and syncope
- "Coat-hanger" neck and shoulder discomfort
- Cognitive slowing when upright
- Headache
- Visual graying
- Dyspnea
- Angina
- Tremulousness
- Leg muscle weakness
- Falls

General symptoms (in any posture)
- Fatigue
- Weakness
- Nausea
- Urinary frequency
- Nocturia
- Constipation (can be severe)
- Loss of sweating (may be patchy)
- Heat intolerance

sudomotor axonal reflex test or a thermoregulatory sweat test).[30] Quantitative sudomotor axonal reflex test involves the iontophoresis of acetylcholine at different locations in the arm and leg to assess the ability of that region to sweat when provoked (intact reflex is present), whereas the thermoregulatory sweat test determines if and where a person sweats in response to environmental heating. The sympathetic noradrenergic nervous system is assessed with an orthostatic challenge (5–10 minute head-up tilt) and the continuous beat-to-beat BP response to a Valsalva maneuver, a cold pressor test (hand in ice water for 60 seconds), and an isometric hand grip test.[28,29] Although beat-to-beat assessments of BP can be accomplished with an arterial line, it is more common to use a noninvasive continuous BP system in most autonomic laboratories.

Valsalva maneuver

The Valsalva maneuver can be a very informative test in nOH. During continuous HR and BP monitoring, patients are asked to perform a forced expiratory effort at a standard expiratory pressure of 40 mm Hg for 15 seconds. The BP waveform consists of four well-defined phases. Phases I

and II represent the strain phases, and phases III and IV are in recovery poststrain. Phases I and III deflections are caused by mechanical perturbations and represent changes in intrathoracic pressure at the beginning and the end of the Valsalva maneuver, whereas phases II and IV represent the clinically relevant stages.[31] In healthy individuals, the BP and pulse pressure decrease initially during the strain phase of Valsalva because of diminished venous return (**Fig. 4**A). This hypotension is then sensed by intact baroreceptors, with resultant increased sympathetic tone. This leads to α-adrenergic receptor-mediated vasoconstriction and BP recovery in late phase II. With release of Valsalva, and normalization of venous return, there is an overshoot of BP in phase IV (combination of optimal venous return and vasoconstriction) before the BP returns to baseline.[32]

Patients with nOH are not able to generate an appropriate increase in sympathetically mediated vasoconstriction in response to the initial hypotension. They typically lack the late phase II BP recovery and the phase IV BP overshoot (see **Fig. 4**B). Rather, the BP slowly drifts back up to baseline after the Valsalva-induced hypotension.

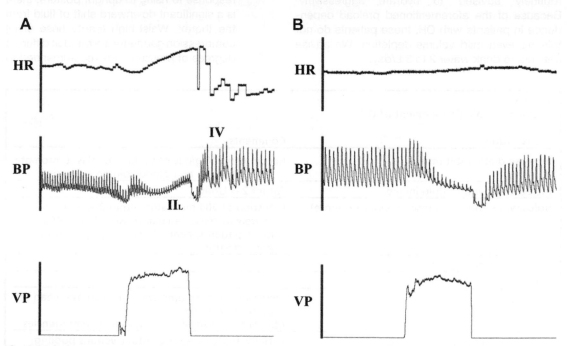

Fig. 4. Valsalva maneuver. During the Valsalva maneuver, the patient is asked to blow and generate approximately 40 mm Hg of Valsalva pressure (VP) for 15 seconds while continuously monitoring HR and BP. In a healthy individual (*A*), the BP and pulse pressure initially decease because of the drop in venous return, but this hypotension triggers an increase in sympathoneurally mediated vasoconstriction. The BP starts to recover in late phase II (II_L). After release of VP (and with it increased venous return) the BP overshoots in phase IV (IV) before returning to baseline. A patient with nOH (*B*) might not be able to generate the appropriate sympathoneurally mediated vasoconstriction in response to the initial hypotension. Patients with nOH typically lack the late phase II BP recovery and the phase IV BP overshoot.

Treatment of nOH

Treatment for nOH is largely empiric with only poor evidence from randomized, placebo-controlled drug trials.[33] Patients who are asymptomatic may require no treatment, although they should be followed clinically for the development of symptoms. Symptomatic patients, however, can be treated with nonpharmacologic (**Table 3**) and pharmacologic (**Table 4**) measures.

Nonpharmacologic Therapy for nOH

Medication withdrawal

In many cases, nOH can be made worse (or converted from asymptomatic to symptomatic) by prescribed medications (see **Table 3**). The BP of patients with nOH is very preload-dependent, so patients with nOH are exquisitely sensitive to diuretics and venodilators (e.g., nitrates). These medications should be withdrawn whenever possible. Direct vasodilators, including α-adrenergic antagonists (e.g., tamsulosin), are commonly used to treat benign prostatic hypertrophy. These agents worsen orthostatic hypotension, or even induce syncope in some individuals. Patients are routinely advised to hydrate aggressively. Because of the aforementioned preload dependence in patients with OH, these patients do not tolerate even mild volume depletion. We advise patients to drink water 2 to 3 L/day.

Postural maneuvers in nOH

The following postural maneuvers are useful in nOH:

- Elevate head of bed: Renal perfusion pressure is often highest at night because of the higher supine BPs that these patients experience compared with seated or standing BPs during the day. This can lead to more nocturnal urine production and subsequently a nocturnal reduction in blood volume, resulting in worsened orthostatic hypotension on awaking in the morning. This problem can be blunted by elevating the head of the bed (effectively tilting the patient) at night, similar to the strategy used in patients with gastroesophageal reflux disease.
- Physical counterpressure maneuvers: Patients should be encouraged to use physical countermeasures, such as standing up slowly and contracting the calf muscles while standing to encourage venous return from the legs. These easy changes can be effective maneuvers when orthostatic hypotension is not overly severe.
- Waist-high compression stockings: In response to rising to upright posture, there is a significant downward shift of fluid from the thorax. Waist-high (panty hose style) compression garments are rated at different degrees of pressure. It is recommended to

---

Table 3
Nonpharmacologic treatment of OH

Intervention	Comments
Increase dietary salt intake	Recommend 10 g/day of sodium; goal is to promote fluid retention and blood volume expansion
Increase water and fluid intake	Target 2–3 L/day
Bolus water ingestion (osmopressor response)	Ingestion of 500 mL water within 2–3 min can acutely increase vascular resistance and BP in many patients; peak effect is between 20–40 min postingestion
Caffeinated beverages	
Physical maneuvers	
• Leg crossing	Increases standing time and may increase mean BP by 10–15 mm Hg
• Squatting	May prevent loss of consciousness in emergencies
External pressure to lower body • Bandages firmly wrapped around the legs • Snugly fitted abdominal binders • Waist-high compression garments	• Helps to decrease orthostatic venous pooling • Most venous pooling occurs in abdomen • Can be uncomfortable to wear (hot and itchy) and require help to put on in elderly patients • Start with 30–40 mm Hg pressure for compression garments • It can be difficult to adequately tighten abdominal binders

Table 4
Pharmacologic treatment for OH

Drug	Dose	Mechanism of Action	Adverse Effect	Comments
Midodrine	2.5–10 mg PO q4h x 3/d; can be taken on PRN basis	α_1-Adrenergic receptor agonist with vasoconstriction	Supine hypertension, piloerection, urinary retention, scalp itch/ irritation	FDA- approved agent for treatment of nOH Midodrine should not be taken within 4 h of lying down
Fludrocortisone	0.05–0.2 mg PO daily	Fluorinated corticosteroid with affinity for the mineralocorticoid receptors; leads to increased renal Na^+ retention, K^+ excretion, and increased extracellular fluid retention	Supine hypertension, headache, hypokalemia, cardiac edema	Must follow serum potassium with chronic use, and may require potassium replacement Can worsen supine hypertension
Yohimbine	5.4–10.8 mg PO TID	α_2-Adrenergic receptor antagonist, with increased sympathoneural tone	Irritability, hypertension, anxiety, scalp itch	Although FDA approved, it is no longer manufactured Available through compounding pharmacies
Pyridostigmine	30–60 mg PO TID	Acetylcholinesterase inhibitor that prolongs acetylcholine effect in autonomic ganglia to increase sympathetic tone	Excessive salivation, increased peristalsis, nausea and vomiting	Maximal effect seen when upright vs supine Can also help with chronic constipation
Caffeine/ergotamine combination	100 mg/1 mg PO 1 tablet BID	Antagonizes vasodilatory effects of endogenous adenosine	Supine hypertension	Cannot use adenosine for SVT termination
Octreotide	12.5–50 µg SQ BID	Somatostatin analogue that induces splanchnic vasoconstriction	Severe seated hypertension	Peptide that requires refrigeration and multiple daily injections (like insulin)
Erythropoietin	25–50 units/kg SQ 3/wk	Stimulates red blood cell production	Hypertension, polycythemia	Can worsen supine hypertension Iron supplements required Must follow hematocrit carefully

Abbreviations: BID, twice per day; FDA, US Food and Drug Administration; nOH, neurogenic orthostatic hypotension; PO, per os; PRN, as needed; SQ, subcutaneous administration; SVT, supraventricular tachycardia; TID, three times per day.

start with 30 to 40 mm Hg of compression to augment venous return.[34] This can be too tight for some older patients to don these garments without assistance.

- Abdominal binders: Most of the pooled blood with standing resides in the abdomen rather than the legs.[35] Studies have shown a benefit to compression of the abdomen only with an abdominal binder.[36] However, it can be difficult to tighten the abdominal binder enough to generate a significant amount of abdominal pressure.

The osmopressor response and nOH

In 1999, Jordan and colleagues[37,38] first reported that rapid ingestion of approximately 500 mL of water by patients with nOH resulted in a subacute increase in systolic BP (>40 mm Hg on average). This pressor response peaks between 20 and 40 minutes postingestion. The pressor response relates to the oral ingestion, and not primarily blood volume expansion, because when 500 mL of D5W was given intravenously in the same patients, the BP increase was blunted.[38] The pressor response was only half as strong when patients with nOH drank salt water compared with plain water, suggesting that the water's hypoosmolality may be critical to this response.[39] The BP increase is mediated by the sympathetic nervous system.[38] The authors advise their patients to drink 500 mL of water rapidly (over 2 minutes) in the morning about 10 minutes before getting out of bed.

Pharmacologic Treatment of nOH

The pharmacologic therapy of nOH involves one of two main strategies: to expand the blood volume and to use short-acting pressor agents (see **Table 4**). The former raises the BP during day and night, whereas the latter raises the BP for a few hours during the period when the patient is upright (and needing BP support).

Volume expansion

Two methods of volume expansion are fludrocortisone and recombinant erythropoietin (EPO). Fludrocortisone promotes increased renal sodium reabsorption and ideally increases intravascular volume. Because fludrocortisone increases daytime and nighttime BP, it can exacerbate supine hypertension in susceptible individuals. Patients with severe autonomic failure may also have anemia. EPO could help with blood volume repletion and correction of symptomatic anemia. Biaggioni and colleagues[40] showed that EPO use in patients with nOH improved standing BP and symptoms, but also noted that use was limited by exaggerated supine hypertension in some patients.

Short-acting pressor agents

Short-acting pressor agents include the following:

- Midodrine: This is the only medication approved by the US Food and Drug Administration for the treatment of nOH. The metabolite is a vasoconstrictor and a venoconstrictor by α_1-adrenoreceptor agonism. A pill starts working within 20 to 30 minutes and the effect lasts for about 4 hours. The patient should be instructed not to lie down within 4 hours of a dose. Midodrine should be started at 2.5 mg orally every 4 hours x 3/day, but can safely be increased to 10 mg/dose.
- Yohimbine: This is an α_2-adrenergic receptor antagonist. α_2-Adrenergic receptors work to decrease sympathetic nervous outflow. By blocking the "brake" on sympathetic outflow, yohimbine facilitates increased sympathetic nervous system activity and unrestrained norepinephrine release from sympathetic neurons, inducing a pressor response to midodrine in patients with OH.[41] Yohimbine (5.4–10.8 mg orally three times a day) is no longer manufactured, but is still available through compounding pharmacies.
- Pyridostigmine: This is a peripheral acetylcholinesterase inhibitor that acts to increase acetylcholine concentrations in the autonomic ganglia. Pyridostigmine (60 mg orally three times a day) modestly reduces the fall in standing BP, but does not increase supine BP.[42,43] Pyridostigmine also increases bowel motility in patients with autonomic failure who are often chronically constipated.
- Norepinephrine reuptake transporter inhibitors: These can increase BP by increasing synaptic norepinephrine in sympathetic neurons. Atomoxetine can significantly increase BP in patients with MSA.[27]
- Cafergot (caffeine, 100 mg, and ergotamine, 1 mg): This causes vasoconstriction through a nonsympathomimetic mechanism.
- Octreotide (12.5–50 µg subcutaneously twice a day): This is an injectable peptide. It likely works through splanchnic vasoconstriction with resultant blood shunting into the central circulation.

Management of Supine Hypertension with nOH

Supine hypertension can often coexist with nOH, and is seen in approximately 60% of patients with nOH assessed at the Vanderbilt Autonomic

Dysfunction Center.[24] In patients with essential hypertension, sustained elevated BP is well-recognized to increase cardiovascular morbidity and mortality, but the consequences of chronic supine hypertension are not well documented,[24] with the exception of accelerated renal dysfunction.[44] In addition to long-term cardiovascular damage, patients with nOH with supine hypertension may have inappropriate nocturnal pressure natriuresis that can result in exaggerated volume depletion by early morning, and an exaggeration of morning symptoms.[45] Treatment options for supine hypertension include sleeping with the head of the bed elevated 6 to 9 inches; a sweet desert at bedtime; nitroglycerine patch, 0.1 mg/h on at bedtime (off 10 minutes before getting up, can be titrated up as needed); and hydralazine, 25 to 50 mg orally at bedtime.

SUMMARY

Orthostatic hypotension is an important cause of syncope, especially in the older patients. Although there are multiple causes, the treatments are focused on improving symptoms. The mainstays of therapy are careful attention to hydration; bolus ingestion of water (osmopressor response); and the judicious use of short-acting pressor agents for the orthostatic hypotension. A significant proportion of patients can also have supine hypertension, which may necessitate the use of short-acting pressor agents overnight.

ACKNOWLEDGMENTS

The authors thank Dr David Robertson for his leadership in the field of autonomic disorders, and his training of numerous investigators in the field of autonomic physiology. They also thank Dr Emily M. Garland for her thoughtful review of this manuscript.

REFERENCES

1. Raj SR. The postural tachycardia syndrome (POTS): pathophysiology, diagnosis & management. Indian Pacing Electrophysiol J 2006;6:84–99.
2. Freeman R, Wieling W, Axelrod FB, et al. Consensus statement on the definition of orthostatic hypotension, neurally mediated syncope and the postural tachycardia syndrome. Auton Neurosci 2011;161:46–8.
3. Gehrking JA, Hines SM, Benrud-Larson LM, et al. What is the minimum duration of head-up tilt necessary to detect orthostatic hypotension? Clin Auton Res 2005;15:71–5.
4. Raj SR. What is the optimal orthostatic stress to diagnose orthostatic hypotension? Clin Auton Res 2005;15:67–8.
5. Gibbons CH, Freeman R. Delayed orthostatic hypotension: a frequent cause of orthostatic intolerance. Neurology 2006;67:28–32.
6. Soteriades ES, Evans JC, Larson MG, et al. Incidence and prognosis of syncope. N Engl J Med 2002;347:878–85.
7. Sarasin FP, Louis-Simonet M, Carballo D, et al. Prevalence of orthostatic hypotension among patients presenting with syncope in the ED. Am J Emerg Med 2002;20:497–501.
8. Rutan GH, Hermanson B, Bild DE, et al. Orthostatic hypotension in older adults. The Cardiovascular Health Study. CHS Collaborative Research Group. Hypertension 1992;19:508–19.
9. Shibao C, Grijalva CG, Raj SR, et al. Orthostatic hypotension-related hospitalizations in the United States. Am J Med 2007;120:975–80.
10. Fagard RH, De CP. Orthostatic hypotension is a more robust predictor of cardiovascular events than nighttime reverse dipping in elderly. Hypertension 2010;56:56–61.
11. Vernino S, Low PA, Fealey RD, et al. Autoantibodies to ganglionic acetylcholine receptors in autoimmune autonomic neuropathies. N Engl J Med 2000;343:847–55.
12. Hollenbeck R, Black BK, Peltier AC, et al. Long-term treatment with rituximab of autoimmune autonomic ganglionopathy in a patient with lymphoma. Arch Neurol 2011;68:372–5.
13. Schroeder C, Vernino S, Birkenfeld AL, et al. Plasma exchange for primary autoimmune autonomic failure. N Engl J Med 2005;353:1585–90.
14. Gibbons CH, Vernino SA, Freeman R. Combined immunomodulatory therapy in autoimmune autonomic ganglionopathy. Arch Neurol 2008;65:213–7.
15. Schrag A, Ben-Shlomo Y, Quinn NP. Prevalence of progressive supranuclear palsy and multiple system atrophy: a cross-sectional study. Lancet 1999;354:1771–5.
16. Vanacore N, Bonifati V, Fabbrini G, et al. Epidemiology of multiple system atrophy. ESGAP Consortium. European Study Group on Atypical Parkinsonisms. Neurol Sci 2001;22:97–9.
17. Parikh SM, Diedrich A, Biaggioni I, et al. The nature of the autonomic dysfunction in multiple system atrophy. J Neurol Sci 2002;200:1–10.
18. Wenning GK, Geser F, Stampfer-Kountchev M, et al. Multiple system atrophy: an update. Mov Disord 2003;18(Suppl 6):S34–42.
19. Bower JH, Maraganore DM, McDonnell SK, et al. Incidence of progressive supranuclear palsy and multiple system atrophy in Olmsted County, Minnesota, 1976 to 1990. Neurology 1997;49:1284–8.

20. Schrag A, Wenning GK, Quinn N, et al. Survival in multiple system atrophy. Mov Disord 2008;23: 294–6.

21. Gilman S, Wenning GK, Low PA, et al. Second consensus statement on the diagnosis of multiple system atrophy. Neurology 2008;71:670–6.

22. Ozawa T, Healy DG, Abou-Sleiman PM, et al. The alpha-synuclein gene in multiple system atrophy. J Neurol Neurosurg Psychiatry 2006;77:464–7.

23. Papp MI, Kahn JE, Lantos PL. Glial cytoplasmic inclusions in the CNS of patients with multiple system atrophy (striatonigral degeneration, olivo-pontocerebellar atrophy and Shy-Drager syndrome). J Neurol Sci 1989;94:79–100.

24. Shibao C, Gamboa A, Diedrich A, et al. Management of hypertension in the setting of autonomic failure: a pathophysiological approach. Hypertension 2005;45:469–76.

25. Tipre DN, Goldstein DS. Cardiac and extracardiac sympathetic denervation in Parkinson's disease with orthostatic hypotension and in pure autonomic failure. J Nucl Med 2005;46:1775–81.

26. Bradbury S, Eggleston C. Postural hypotension with syncope: a report of three cases. Am Heart J 1925; 1:75–86.

27. Shibao C, Raj SR, Gamboa A, et al. Norepinephrine transporter blockade with atomoxetine induces hypertension in patients with impaired autonomic function. Hypertension 2007;50:47–53.

28. Freeman R. Clinical practice. Neurogenic orthostatic hypotension. N Engl J Med 2008;358:615–24.

29. Mosqueda-Garcia R. Evaluation of autonomic failure. In: Robertson D, Biaggioni I, editors. Disorders of the autonomic nervous system. Luxembourg: Harwood Academic Publishers GmbH; 1995. p. 25–59.

30. Low VA, Sandroni P, Fealey RD, et al. Detection of small-fiber neuropathy by sudomotor testing. Muscle Nerve 2006;34:57–61.

31. Raj SR, Robertson D, Biaggioni I, et al. Abnormal valsalva maneuver is not always a sign of congestive heart failure. Am J Med 2007;120:e15–6.

32. Sandroni P. Clinical evaluation of autonomic disorders. In: Robertson D, Biaggioni I, Burnstock G, et al, editors. Primer on the autonomic nervous system. 3rd edition. San Diego: Academic press; 2012. p. 377–82.

33. Logan IC, Witham MD. Efficacy of treatments for orthostatic hypotension: a systematic review. Age Ageing 2012;41:587–94.

34. Podoleanu C, Maggi R, Brignole M, et al. Lower limb and abdominal compression bandages prevent progressive orthostatic hypotension in elderly persons: a randomized single-blind controlled study. J Am Coll Cardiol 2006;48:1425–32.

35. Diedrich A, Biaggioni I. Segmental orthostatic fluid shifts. Clin Auton Res 2004;14:146–7.

36. Smit AA, Wieling W, Fujimura J, et al. Use of lower abdominal compression to combat orthostatic hypotension in patients with autonomic dysfunction. Clin Auton Res 2004;14:167–75.

37. Jordan J, Shannon JR, Grogan E, et al. A potent pressor response elicited by drinking water. Lancet 1999;353:723.

38. Jordan J, Shannon JR, Black BK, et al. The pressor response to water drinking in humans: a sympathetic reflex? Circulation 2000;101:504–9.

39. Raj SR, Biaggioni I, Black BK, et al. Sodium paradoxically reduces the gastropressor response in patients with orthostatic hypotension. Hypertension 2006;48:329–34.

40. Biaggioni I, Robertson D, Krantz S, et al. The anemia of primary autonomic failure and its reversal with recombinant erythropoietin. Ann Intern Med 1994;121: 181–6.

41. Jordan J, Shannon JR, Biaggioni I, et al. Contrasting actions of pressor agents in severe autonomic failure. Am J Med 1998;105:116–24.

42. Singer W, Sandroni P, Opfer-Gehrking TL, et al. Pyridostigmine treatment trial in neurogenic orthostatic hypotension. Arch Neurol 2006;63:513–8.

43. Shibao C, Okamoto LE, Gamboa A, et al. Comparative efficacy of yohimbine against pyridostigmine for the treatment of orthostatic hypotension in autonomic failure. Hypertension 2010;56:847–51.

44. Garland EM, Gamboa A, Okamoto L, et al. Renal impairment of pure autonomic failure. Hypertension 2009;54:1057–61.

45. Blanker MH, Bernsen RM, Ruud Bosch JL, et al. Normal values and determinants of circadian urine production in older men: a population based study. J Urol 2002;168:1453–7.

Confounders of Vasovagal Syncope
Postural Tachycardia Syndrome

Victor C. Nwazue, MD[a,b], Satish R. Raj, MD, MSCI[a,b],*

KEYWORDS

- Syncope • Vasovagal • Postural tachycardia syndrome • Treatment • Autonomic dysfunction
- Vasovagal syncope • Blood pressure • Heart rate

KEY POINTS

- A common confounder of vasovagal syncope and presyncope is postural tachycardia syndrome (POTS), a multisystem disorder of the autonomic nervous system.
- The hallmark manifestation of POTS is symptomatic orthostatic tachycardia, with lightheadedness and presyncope.
- Patients with POTS have a heart rate increase of 30 bpm or more with standing (within 10 minutes), often have high levels of upright plasma norepinephrine, and often have a low blood volume.
- POTS can often be differentiated from vasovagal syncope by its hemodynamic pattern during tilt table test and differing clinical characteristics.
- Exercise training has been found to be highly effective at improving the physiology and symptoms in patients with POTS. Pharmacologic therapies aimed at correcting the hypovolemia and the excess sympathetic tone may also help improve the symptoms.

INTRODUCTION

Although most cases of syncope are caused by vasovagal syncope (VVS), more common than syncope is presyncope. Cardiologists working in a syncope clinic or in a tilt table laboratory realize that a common confounder of VVS and presyncope is postural tachycardia syndrome (POTS; primarily presenting with presyncope). **Table 1** highlights some contrasting clinical characteristics between these 2 disorders. These disorders can

have distinct hemodynamic patterns during tilt table testing. During head-up tilt:

- Patients with VVS often hold a steady blood pressure (BP) for several minutes (often >10 minutes) post head-up tilt, before they develop symptoms and decrease their BP rapidly (**Fig. 1**A).
- Patients with POTS do not usually decrease their BP with head-up tilt. Rather, they classically have an excessive increase in their

Research funding: Supported in part by National Institutes of Health grants R01 HL102387, P01 HL56693, and UL1 TR000445 (Clinical and Translational Science Award).

Conflicts of interest: None.

[a] Division of Clinical Pharmacology, Department of Medicine, Autonomic Dysfunction Center, Vanderbilt University School of Medicine, AA3228 Medical Center North, 1161 21st Avenue South, Nashville, TN 37232-2195, USA;

[b] Division of Clinical Pharmacology, Department of Pharmacology, Autonomic Dysfunction Center, Vanderbilt University School of Medicine, AA3228 Medical Center North, 1161 21st Avenue South, Nashville, TN 37232-2195, USA

* Corresponding author. Division of Clinical Pharmacology, Departments of Medicine & Pharmacology, Autonomic Dysfunction Center, Vanderbilt University School of Medicine, AA3228 Medical Center North, 1161 21st Avenue South, Nashville, TN 37232-2195.

E-mail address: satish.raj@vanderbilt.edu

Cardiol Clin 31 (2013) 101–109

http://dx.doi.org/10.1016/j.ccl.2012.09.004

Table 1
Clinical comparison of VVS and POTS

Features	VVS	POTS
Typical age	Any age; first episode usually in second/third decade	13–50 y
Gender (% female)	60	85
Symptoms with body position change	After prolonged sitting or standing	Immediately with sitting or standing
Syncope	+++	±
Presyncope	+	++++
Orthostatic hypotension	± (usually only at time of faint)	±
Hemodynamic pattern with head-up tilt	Sudden decrease in BP and HR	Early increase in HR ≥30 bpm

Abbreviations: BP, blood pressure; HR, heart rate.

heart rate (HR) (see **Fig. 1**B). This article reviews the presentation, putative pathophysiology, investigation approach, and treatment of POTS.

HEMODYNAMIC PHYSIOLOGY OF STANDING: HEALTHY AND POTS

With the assumption of an upright posture, there is a downward shift of ∼500 mL of blood to the dependent areas (mainly abdomen and legs). This gravitational shift in blood results in decreased venous return, decreased cardiac output, and decreased BP (**Fig. 2**A).[1] This situation unloads the baroreceptors, and triggers a reflex sympathetic activation, with a resultant increase in HR and systemic vasoconstriction (countering the initial decline in BP). In a healthy individual, the net effect of assumption of upright posture is an increase in HR of 10 to 20 bpm, a minimal change in systolic BP, and a ∼5-mm Hg increase in diastolic BP.

In patients with POTS (see **Fig. 2**B), the initial response to upright posture can include a profound decrease in stroke volume. With engagement of the baroreflex, there can be a vigorous increase in sympathetic tone and an exaggerated increase in HR. The BP may remain unchanged or even increase if there is excessive sympathetically mediated vasoconstriction. Presyncope can result from the excessive tachycardia or the increased sympathoneural tone.

POTS

Patients with POTS have an excessive increase in HR in response to upright posture (in the absence of orthostatic hypotension) with improvement in symptoms on lying down.[1,2]

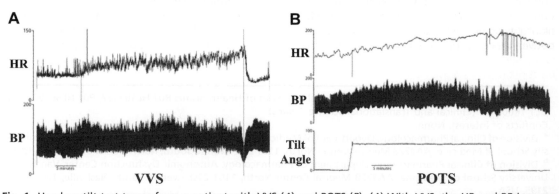

Fig. 1. Head-up tilt test traces from a patient with VVS (*A*) and POTS (*B*). (*A*) With VVS, the HR and BP increase a little at the onset of tilt, and they are maintained for more than 25 minutes before a sudden precipitous decrease in BP before the table is returned to the supine position. (*B*) With POTS, the BP often increases a little with head-up tilt, and starts to return to baseline when the table returns to the supine position. (*Reprinted from* Raj SR, Sheldon RS. Head-up tilt-table test. In: Saksena S, Camm AJ, editors. Electrophysiological disorders of the heart. 2nd edition. New York: Saunders; 2012. p. 73–6-73–8; with permission.)

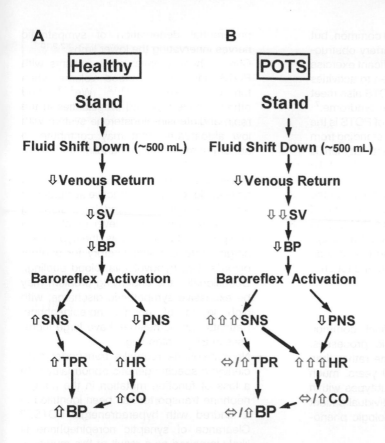

A

Healthy

Stand
↓
Fluid Shift Down (~500 mL)
↓
⇩Venous Return
↓
⇩SV
↓
⇩BP
↓
Baroreflex Activation
↙   ↘
⇧SNS   ⇩PNS
↙   ↘   ↓
⇧TPR   ⇧HR
↓
⇧CO
↓
⇧BP

B

POTS

Stand
↓
Fluid Shift Down (~500 mL)
↓
⇩Venous Return
↓
⇩⇩SV
↓
⇩BP
↓
Baroreflex Activation
↙   ↘
⇧⇧⇧SNS   ⇩PNS
↙   ↘   ↓
⇔/⇧TPR   ⇧⇧⇧HR
↓
⇔/⇧CO
↓
⇔/⇧BP

Fig. 2. Physiology of standing in a healthy individual and patient with POTS. (*A*) With the assumption of an upright posture in a healthy individual, there is a downward shift of ~500 mL of blood with a decrease in venous return, stroke volume (*SV*) and eventually BP.[1] This situation unloads the baroreceptors and triggers reflex sympathetic nervous system (*SNS*) activation, with a resultant increase in HR and systemic vasoconstriction (countering the initial decline in BP). In a healthy individual, the net effect of assumption of upright posture is an increase in HR of 10 to 20 bpm, a minimal change in systolic BP, and a ~5-mm Hg increase in diastolic BP. (*B*) In patients with POTS, the initial response to upright posture can include a profound decrease in SV. With engagement of the baroreflex, there can be a vigorous increase in SNS tone and an exaggerated increase in HR. The BP may remain unchanged or even increase if there is excessive SNS-mediated vasoconstriction. Presyncope can result from the excessive HR increase or the increased SNS tone. CO, cardiac output; PNS, parasympathetic nervous system; TPR, total peripheral resistance.

It is estimated that there are ~500,000 Americans diagnosed with POTS in the United States,[3] with 80% to 90% female patients,[1,4,5] often of childbearing age.[1,6]

POTS DIAGNOSTIC CRITERIA

POTS is defined as the presence of symptoms of orthostatic intolerance for more than 6 months accompanied by an HR increase of 30 bpm or greater within 10 minutes of assuming an upright posture in the absence of orthostatic hypotension (decrease in BP >20/10 mm Hg). The syndrome must occur in the absence of prolonged bed rest, medications that impair autonomic regulation (eg, diuretics, vasodilators, diuretics, sympatholytics, or certain antidepressants), or any other chronic debilitating disorders that might cause tachycardia (such as dehydration, anemia, or hyperthyroidism). Orthostatic tachycardia is necessary, but not sufficient to make the diagnosis of POTS; typical symptoms are also required (**Box 1**).

POTS CLINICAL FEATURES

Symptoms in patients with POTS include lightheadedness, shortness of breath, palpitations, tremulousness, chest discomfort, headache, visual disturbances, mental clouding (brain fog), and nausea. Only some (~30%) patients with POTS have frank syncope, but daily or almost daily

---

Box 1
Diagnostic criteria for POTS

- HR increase 30 bpm or greater from lying to standing
- Absence of significant decrease in BP with standing
- Positional symptoms
  - Many symptoms are worse with upright posture and improve on lying down
  - Some symptoms can be nonpositional (eg, fatigue, headache)
- Chronic symptoms
  - Duration 6 months or longer
- Absence of other overt cause for tachycardia
  - For example, acute blood loss, prolonged bedrest, hyperthyroidism, tachycardia-promoting medications

presyncope occurs. Chest pains are common, but almost never caused by coronary artery obstruction. Most patients complain of significant exercise intolerance and extreme fatigue, even to activities of daily living. Some patients with POTS also meet diagnostic criteria for chronic fatigue syndrome.[7]

The most striking physical feature of POTS is the severe tachycardia that develops on standing from a supine position. Recent data suggest that there is a significant circadian variability in the orthostatic tachycardia in patients with POTS, with greater orthostatic tachycardia in the morning than in the evening.[8] Another remarkable physical feature of POTS is the dependent acrocyanosis that occurs in close to 50% of patients with POTS (**Fig. 3**).[1] These patients experience a dark red-blue discoloration of their legs, which are cold to the touch.

POTS PATHOPHYSIOLOGY

Tachycardia on standing is a final common pathway of many pathophysiologic processes. POTS is a heterogeneous syndrome rather than a single disease. Over the last 20 years, much has been learned about specific subtypes within POTS, although categorizing the individual patient remains difficult. Some pathophysiologic phenotypes include the following:

- Neuropathic POTS: some patients likely have a form of dysautonomia, with

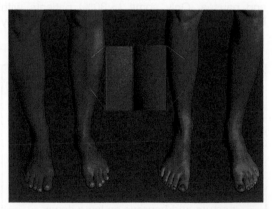

Fig. 3. Acrocyanosis in POTS. A striking physical feature in POTS is the gross change in leg skin color that can occur with standing. The panel shows the legs of a healthy individual (*left*) and a patient with POTS (*right*) who have each been standing for 5 minutes. The patient with POTS (*right*) has significant dark red mottling of her legs extending up to the knees while standing, whereas the healthy individual does not have a similar discoloration. (*Reprinted from* Raj SR. The postural tachycardia syndrome (POTS): pathophysiology, diagnosis & management. Indian Pacing Electrophysiol J 2006;6:88; with permission.)

preferential denervation of sympathetic nerves innervating the lower limbs.[2,9,10]

- Chronic hypovolemia: many patients with POTS have a low blood volume when formally assessed.[4,11,12] We[4,13] and others[14] have reported irregularities in the renin-angiotensin-aldosterone system with low aldosterone that may contribute to abnormal renal sodium handling and hypovolemia in POTS.

- Hyperadrenergic POTS: many patients have evidence of a hyperactive sympathetic nervous system, indicated by a standing plasma norepinephrine level greater than 600 pg/mL.[6] In most cases, the hyperadrenergic state is compensatory for another disorder (eg, hypovolemia, blood pooling). Occasionally, the underlying problem may be excessive sympathetic discharge, with high levels of upright norepinephrine. Patients can sometimes have large increases in BP on standing.

- Norepinephrine reuptake transporter deficiency: a specific genetic abnormality with a loss of function mutation in the norepinephrine transporter has been identified in a kindred with hyperadrenergic POTS.[15] Clearance of synaptic norepinephrine is likely impaired as a result of this mutation. Many psychiatric drugs inhibit the norepinephrine reuptake transporter, recreating an orthostatic tachycardia phenotype in previously unaffected patients.[16,17]

- Mast cell activation disorder: some patients with POTS have mast cell degranulation without an overt trigger. These patients have episodic flushing and abnormal increases in urine methylhistamine (the primary urinary metabolite of histamine).[18]

INVESTIGATION OF POTS

- Orthostatic challenge: POTS diagnostic criteria require an increase in HR of 30 bpm or greater within 10 minutes of upright posture (tilt or standing, even although these are not identical (**Table 2**).[19]

- Confirm sinus tachycardia: patients with POTS should have only sinus tachycardia. An electrocardiogram should be performed routinely to rule out the presence of an accessory bypass tract or any abnormalities of cardiac conduction. A Holter monitor might prove useful to exclude a reentrant dysrhythmia, especially if the patient gives a history of paroxysmal tachycardia with a sudden onset and offset.

Table 2
Diagnostic tests in POTS

Diagnostic Test	Comments
Orthostatic challenge	Increase in HR ≥30 bpm within 10 min of upright posture required for diagnosis
Electrocardiogram/cardiac monitoring	Rule out any abnormal cardiac conduction; confirm sinus (and not ectopic) tachycardia
Echocardiogram	Rule out structural heart abnormalities
Supine and upright plasma NE	Plasma NE ≥600 pg/mL suggestive of a hyperadrenergic response
Autonomic function test	Intact (and sometimes vigorous) HR and BP recovery with Valsalva
Blood volume assessment	A significant proportion of patients with POTS have low blood volume
Other blood test: hemogram, electrolytes, thyroid function, celiac panel, vitamin B_{12}, and serum iron panel	To rule other medical conditions that can promote sinus tachycardia

Abbreviation: NE, norepinephrine.

- Echocardiogram: required in individual cases when there is doubt about the structural integrity of the heart.
- Supine and upright plasma norepinephrine: the supine norepinephrine is often high normal in patients with POTS, and the upright norepinephrine is usually increased (>600 pg/mL). This situation likely reflects the exaggerated sympathoneural tone that is present in many patients while upright.
- Autonomic function tests: responses are usually intact or exaggerated to both cardiovagal testing (sinus arrhythmia), and Valsalva BP in phase II and IV.
- Blood volume assessment: the blood volume is low in many patients with POTS,[4] and this can be assessed in many nuclear medicine laboratories.
- Blood tests: complete blood count and electrolyte panel; thyroid function tests, celiac panel with gastrointestinal symptoms, vitamin B_{12}, and iron indices.

NONPHARMACOLOGIC TREATMENT OF POTS

- Remove potentially contributory medications: especially venodilators (such as nitrates), diuretics, and norepinephrine reuptake transporter-inhibiting drugs (**Table 3**).
- Reconditioning: patients who have been sedentary or in bed for prolonged periods of time require reconditioning.
- Avoid ablating the sinus node: although there are anecdotal reports of benefits

with sinus node modification, many patients do poorly after procedure (potentially with a pacemaker). The underlying problem is not in the sinus node.
- Patient education: patients should learn to avoid aggravating factors such as dehydration (drink 8–10 cups of water/d and consume ~200 mEq Na^+/d) and extreme heat. There are many patient Web sites, include the Vanderbilt autonomic dysfunction site (http://www.mc.vanderbilt.edu/gcec/adc).
- Waist-high compression garments: 30 to 40 mm Hg of counterpressure can minimize venous pooling, especially when the patient needs to stand for prolonged periods. These garments can be hot, itchy, and uncomfortable.

Intravenous Saline for POTS

Acute blood volume expansion with intravenous saline 1 to 2 L is effective at controlling the HR and acutely improving symptoms.[20] Because of vascular access issues, this treatment is not practical on a day-to-day basis, but can be used as a rescue medicine at times of decompensation.

Exercise Training for POTS

Exercise has routinely been recommended as a part of the POTS treatment regimen for many years. Patients with POTS report feeling debilitated for days after exertion, limiting compliance with exercise training. Anecdotally, patients who did exercise seemed to have a better long-term

Table 3
Nonpharmacologic treatment of POTS

Measures	Mechanism	Comments
Exercise training	Blood volume expansion and reverses cardiac deconditioning	Improves quality of life and physiology (if patient can complete exercise program)
Physical maneuvers		
Squatting	Enhances venous return	May prevent syncope
Sit with feet folded up	Prevents blood pooling	May prevent syncope
Waist-high compression garments	Prevents blood pooling	Start with 30–40 mm Hg pressure for compression garments; can be uncomfortable (hot and itchy) and unfashionable
Aggressive fluid intake	Blood volume expansion	8–10 cups of water/d
Increased sodium intake	Blood volume expansion	Up to 200 mEq Na^+/d
Saline intravenously 1–2 L as needed	Blood volume expansion	Rescue therapy for decompensation

prognosis, but it was not certain if this was a selection bias. Fu and colleagues[21] have recently shown the dramatic benefits of exercise. They administered a structured 3-month exercise program to 19 patients with POTS, and showed improved quality of life, reduced orthostatic tachycardia, and increased blood volume, stroke volume, and left ventricular mass. This study shows that exercise training is an important treatment in this population. Recommendations regarding exercise training for patients with POTS are included in **Box 2**.

PHARMACOLOGIC TREATMENT OF POTS
Volume Expansion

- Fludrocortisone 0.05 to 0.2 mg daily: many patients with POTS are hypovolemic,[4] so fludrocortisone (an aldosterone analogue) is often used. Through enhanced renal sodium retention, it should expand the plasma volume (although the data are poor). Potassium wasting can result in hypokalemia, so serum K^+ should be monitored periodically (**Table 4**).
- Desmopressin 0.2 mg by mouth as needed (not daily): Oral desmopressin promotes renal free water retention, and is often used for enuresis. Desmopressin can acutely lower standing HR in POTS and improve symptoms.[22] Potential side effects include hyponatremia, edema, and headache. Serum Na^+ should be monitored periodically during therapy.

Box 2
Fu/Levine exercise training protocol for patients with POTS

Initial Exercise Training

Avoid upright exercises

Recommend using a rowing machine, recumbent cycle, or swimming.

Intensity: target HR equivalent to 75% to 80% of maximum steady state.

Duration: 3 or 4 sessions/wk for 30 to 45 min/session.

Exercise Training Months 2 to 3

Can begin upright exercise using upright bike, walking, treadmill, or jogging

Intensity: gradually increase intensity to maximal steady state 1/wk and then 2/wk.

Duration: increase as patient becomes fit, with goal of 5 to 6 hours per week.

Resistance Training

Focus on lower body

Start 1/wk for 15 to 20 min/session

Gradually increase to 2/wk for 45 min/session

Long-Term Exercise Training

Patients encouraged to continue exercise indefinitely

Adapted from Fu Q, Vangundy TB, Shibata S, et al. Exercise training versus propranolol in the treatment of the postural orthostatic tachycardia syndrome. Hypertension 2011;58:167–75.

Table 4
Pharmacologic treatment of POTS

Drug	Dose	Mechanism	Adverse Effects	Comments
Propranolol	10–20 mg PO QID	β-Adrenergic receptor antagonist	Bradycardia, hypotension, and bronchospasm	Attenuates symptomatic tachycardia on standing; low doses can help; high doses not tolerated
Pyridostigmine	30–60 mg PO TID	Acetylcholinesterase inhibitor	Abdominal cramping: diarrhea; increased sweating	Attenuates tachycardia and improve symptoms; can be combined with propranolol
Fludrocortisone	0.05–0.2 mg PO daily	Blood volume expansion; synthetic aldosterone	Hypertension, fluid retention, and hypokalemia	Most effective when combined with increased dietary salt and water
Midodrine	2.5–10 mg PO every 4 h TID	Vasoconstriction; α_1 adrenergic receptor agonist	Scalp itch, piloerection, urinary retention, and hypertension	Can improve venous return and decrease reflex tachycardia
Desmopressin (DDAVP)	0.2 mg PO occasionally	Acute blood volume expansion	Water retention; hyponatremia	Follow serum [Na$^+$] carefully
Methyldopa	125 mg PO QHS or BID	Central sympatholytic False neurotransmitter	Sedation and hypotension	Reduce plasma norepinephrine
Clonidine	0.05–0.2 mg BID (or use a long-acting patch)	Central sympatholytic α_2 receptor agonist	Worsens fatigue; sedation and hypotension	Reduce plasma norepinephrine

Abbreviations: BID, twice per day; PO, by mouth; QHS, at bedtime; QID, 4 times per day; TID, 3 times per day.

Sympatholysis

- Propranolol 10 to 20 mg by mouth 4 times a day: many patients report intolerance to β-blockers when first seen at the Vanderbilt Autonomic Dysfunction Center. However, most patients with POTS respond well hemodynamically and symptomatically to low doses of propranolol.[5] More complete β-blockade with higher doses of propranolol causes symptoms to worsen. Long-acting propranolol was not found to be helpful.[14] Propranolol is our first-line pharmacologic agent.
- Methyldopa 125 mg at bedtime or twice a day: methyldopa is a false neurotransmitter that can lower central sympathetic tone. It is particularly useful in hyperadrenergic patients.
- Clonidine 0.05 to 0.2 mg by mouth twice a day (or a long-acting patch): α_2 adrenergic

agonist that acts centrally to decrease sympathetic nervous system tone. It can stabilize HR and BP, but it can also cause drowsiness and fatigue and worsen the mental clouding of some patients.

Vasoconstrictor Therapy

- Midodrine 5 to 10 mg by mouth every 4 hours 3 times day: Because a failure of vascular resistance may be an integral part of neuropathic POTS, vasoconstrictors such as midodrine (α_1 agonist) can be used.[23]

Increasing Vagal Tone

- Pyridostigmine 30 to 60 mg by mouth 3 times a day: pyridostigmine is a peripheral acetylcholinesterase inhibitor. By increasing synaptic acetylcholine at both the autonomic ganglia and the peripheral muscarinic parasympathetic receptors, pyridostigmine significantly restrains the HR in response to standing in patients with POTS.[24,25] Pyridostigmine is most effective in combination with low-dose propranolol. Because pyridostigmine enhances bowel motility, it is often not well tolerated in patients with diarrhea-predominant irritable bowel syndrome symptoms.[26]

Vanderbilt Approach to Pharmacotherapy for POTS

In addition to initial nonpharmacologic approaches, and strong advice about an exercise regimen, most patients with POTS require some pharmacotherapy. We often start with low-dose propranolol. If the patient has hypovolemia, then we add in fludrocortisone. As third-line therapy, if the patient is very hyperadrenergic, then we might consider a central sympatholytic; otherwise, midodrine is our third-line agent.

SUMMARY

POTS is a multisystem disorder of the autonomic nervous system. The hallmark manifestation is symptomatic orthostatic tachycardia, with lightheadedness and presyncope. Although it is not primarily a syncopal disorder, a few patients can also have VVS. POTS is associated with substantial functional disability among otherwise healthy people. Patients with POTS show an HR increase of 30 bpm or more with standing (within 10 minutes), often have high levels of upright plasma norepinephrine, and many patients have a low blood volume. Exercise training has been found to be highly effective at improving the physiology and symptoms in patients with POTS. Pharmacologic therapies aimed at correcting the hypovolemia and the excess sympathetic tone may also help improve the symptoms.

ACKNOWLEDGMENTS

We thank Dr David Robertson for his leadership in autonomic disorders, and his training numerous investigators in autonomic physiology. We also thank Dr Emily M Garland for her thoughtful review of this article.

REFERENCES

1. Raj SR. The postural tachycardia syndrome (POTS): pathophysiology, diagnosis & management. Indian Pacing Electrophysiol J 2006;6:84–99.
2. Schondorf R, Low PA. Idiopathic postural orthostatic tachycardia syndrome: an attenuated form of acute pandysautonomia? Neurology 1993;43:132–7.
3. Robertson D. The epidemic of orthostatic tachycardia and orthostatic intolerance. Am J Med Sci 1999;317:75–7.
4. Raj SR, Biaggioni I, Yamhure PC, et al. Renin-aldosterone paradox and perturbed blood volume regulation underlying postural tachycardia syndrome. Circulation 2005;111:1574–82.
5. Raj SR, Black BK, Biaggioni I, et al. Propranolol decreases tachycardia and improves symptoms in the postural tachycardia syndrome: less is more. Circulation 2009;120:725–34.
6. Garland EM, Raj SR, Black BK, et al. The hemodynamic and neurohumoral phenotype of postural tachycardia syndrome. Neurology 2007;69:790–8.
7. Okamoto LE, Raj SR, Peltier A, et al. Neurohumoral and haemodynamic profile in postural tachycardia and chronic fatigue syndromes. Clin Sci (Lond) 2012;122:183–92.
8. Brewster JA, Garland EM, Biaggioni I, et al. Diurnal variability in orthostatic tachycardia: implications for the postural tachycardia syndrome. Clin Sci (Lond) 2012;122:25–31.
9. Streeten DH. Pathogenesis of hyperadrenergic orthostatic hypotension. Evidence of disordered venous innervation exclusively in the lower limbs. J Clin Invest 1990;86:1582–8.
10. Jacob G, Costa F, Shannon JR, et al. The neuropathic postural tachycardia syndrome. N Engl J Med 2000;343:1008–14.
11. Fouad FM, Tadena-Thome L, Bravo EL, et al. Idiopathic hypovolemia. Ann Intern Med 1986;104:298–303.
12. Streeten DH, Thomas D, Bell DS. The roles of orthostatic hypotension, orthostatic tachycardia, and subnormal erythrocyte volume in the pathogenesis of the chronic fatigue syndrome. Am J Med Sci 2000;320:1–8.
13. Mustafa HI, Garland EM, Biaggioni I, et al. Abnormalities of angiotensin regulation in postural tachycardia syndrome. Heart Rhythm 2011;8:422–8.
14. Fu Q, Vangundy TB, Shibata S, et al. Exercise training versus propranolol in the treatment of the postural orthostatic tachycardia syndrome. Hypertension 2011;58:167–75.
15. Shannon JR, Flattem NL, Jordan J, et al. Orthostatic intolerance and tachycardia associated with norepinephrine-transporter deficiency. N Engl J Med 2000;342:541–9.
16. Vincent S, Bieck PR, Garland EM, et al. Clinical assessment of norepinephrine transporter blockade through biochemical and pharmacological profiles. Circulation 2004;109:3202–7.
17. Schroeder C, Tank J, Boschmann M, et al. Selective norepinephrine reuptake inhibition as a human

model of orthostatic intolerance. Circulation 2002; 105:347–53.

18. Shibao C, Arzubiaga C, Roberts LJ, et al. Hyperadrenergic postural tachycardia syndrome in mast cell activation disorders. Hypertension 2005;45: 385–90.

19. Plash WB, Diedrich A, Biaggioni I, et al. Diagnosing postural tachycardia syndrome: comparison of tilt test versus standing hemodynamics. Clin Sci (Lond) 2013;124:109–14.

20. Jacob G, Shannon JR, Black B, et al. Effects of volume loading and pressor agents in idiopathic orthostatic tachycardia. Circulation 1997;96:575–80.

21. Fu Q, Vangundy TB, Galbreath MM, et al. Cardiac origins of the postural orthostatic tachycardia syndrome. J Am Coll Cardiol 2010;55:2858–68.

22. Coffin ST, Black BK, Biaggioni I, et al. Desmopressin acutely decreases tachycardia and improves symptoms in the postural tachycardia syndrome. Heart Rhythm 2012;9:1484–90.

23. Grubb BP, Karas B, Kosinski D, et al. Preliminary observations on the use of midodrine hydrochloride in the treatment of refractory neurocardiogenic syncope. J Interv Card Electrophysiol 1999;3:139–43.

24. Raj SR, Black BK, Biaggioni I, et al. Acetylcholinesterase inhibition improves tachycardia in postural tachycardia syndrome. Circulation 2005;111: 2734–40.

25. Singer W, Opfer-Gehrking TL, Nickander KK, et al. Acetylcholinesterase inhibition in patients with orthostatic intolerance. J Clin Neurophysiol 2006; 23:476–81.

26. Kanjwal K, Karabin B, Sheikh M, et al. Pyridostigmine in the treatment of postural orthostatic tachycardia: a single-center experience. Pacing Clin Electrophysiol 2011;34:750–5.

Carotid Sinus Syndrome

Colette Seifer, FRCP

KEYWORDS

- Carotid sinus hypersensitivity • Syncope • Falls • Pacemaker • Aging

KEY POINTS

- Although carotid sinus hypersensitivity was first reported more than 200 years ago, a complete understanding of this relatively common clinical finding in older patients has proven elusive.
- Evidence exists to support an association between symptoms, particularly syncope, and a hypersensitive response to carotid sinus massage; however, the clinical implication of a high prevalence in asymptomatic healthy older persons is not known.
- A central degenerative process likely underlies the pathophysiology, but this is currently remains unproven.
- Although selected patients have had symptom improvement with treatment, particularly permanent pacing, there is a dearth of randomized controlled trial data to guide management.

Slowing of the pulse in response to carotid artery pressure was first described by Parry in 1799 (**Box 1**).[1] In 1866, Czermak documented hypotension in response to pressure applied over his own carotid artery; this was the first blood pressure recording during carotid sinus stimulation.[2] The physiology of this phenomenon, however, was not elucidated until the 20th century, with the identification of the reflex nature of carotid sinus stimulation.[3,4] Clinical cases of patients with syncope reproduced by applying pressure to the carotid sinus were reported from the 1930s onwards.[5,6] The term hypersensitivity was first used by Roskam to describe a prolonged period of asystole associated with loss of consciousness during carotid sinus pressure.[5] But it was the seminal descriptive and experimental work by Weiss and Baker that definitively delineated the reflex.[7] Theirs was the first description of the correlation of spontaneous symptoms with induced syncope by carotid sinus stimulation. By studying diverse subjects, they furthered the concept of a distinction between a hypersensitive response to carotid sinus massage in asymptomatic and symptomatic persons.

PHYSIOLOGY
Definition

CSH is defined by the heart rate and blood pressure response to carotid sinus massage (CSM). Cardioinhibitory carotid sinus hypersensitivity (CICSH) is diagnosed by a greater than or equal to 3-second pause, while a vasodepressor response (VDCSH) is the reduction in blood pressure of at least 50 mm Hg in the absence of significant bradycardia (**Box 2**). The third subtype, mixed CSH, is diagnosed by the presence of a greater than or equal to 3-second pause along with a decrease in systolic blood pressure of at least 50 mm Hg upon rhythm resumption.[8,9] The origin of the definition of cardioinhibition dates back to work done by Weiss and Baker, as well as Sigler.[7,10] Years later, Franke advanced the absolute value cut-off for reduction in blood pressure, defining a vasodepressor response.[11] The routine availability of continuous methods for measuring beat-to-beat blood pressure in the 1990s has improved insight into blood pressure response to carotid sinus massage.[2]

Arrhythmia Service, Section of Cardiology, St. Boniface Hospital, The University of Manitoba, Y3006, 401 Tache Avenue, Winnipeg, Manitoba R2H 2A6, Canada
E-mail address: cmseifer@sbgh.mb.ca

Cardiol Clin 31 (2013) 111–121
http://dx.doi.org/10.1016/j.ccl.2012.10.002
0733-8651/13/$ – see front matter © 2013 Elsevier Inc. All rights reserved.

The Carotid Sinus Reflex: Physiology

The carotid sinus is a dilated segment of the left and right internal carotid arteries that acts as a high pressure baroreceptor (**Box 3**). These receptors respond to stretching of the arterial wall so that if arterial pressure suddenly rises, the walls of these vessels passively expand, stimulating firing of these receptors. Stimulation of baroreceptors increases vagal activity and inhibits sympathetic activity.[12] If arterial blood pressure suddenly falls, decreased stretch of the arterial walls leads to a decrease in receptor firing.[13] The afferent limb of this reflex transmits impulses from the carotid sinus, glossopharyngeal, and vagus nerves to the brainstem. These nerves terminate in the nucleus tractus solitarii (NTS), located along the length of the medulla oblongata within the dorsal respiratory group (DRG). The NTS divide into a rostral gustatory nucleus and a caudal region of neurons. Many cardiovascular neurons are positioned within the caudal region, near the midline of the nucleus.[14] The efferent limb of the reflex is carried via the sympathetic and parasympathetic (vagus) nerves to the heart and vessels, controlling heart rate and vasomotor tone. Baroreceptors are acutely sensitive to changes in pressure, rapidly discharging during a rise in blood pressure stimulating an increase in vagal activity and an inhibition of sympathetic activity. Resetting

of baroreceptors occurs as the level of blood pressure fluctuates. Early resetting occurs within minutes of a change in pressure, (eg, during a change in posture). Chronic resetting takes place over months, and this results in a decrease in the sensitivity of the reflex.[15]

The Carotid Sinus Reflex: Pathophysiology

CSH is associated with advancing age and coronary artery disease. However, the mechanisms responsible for this hypersensitivity have proven elusive. Atherosclerosis may diminish carotid sinus compliance, resulting in a reduction in afferent impulse traffic in the baroreflex pathway. Although plausible, this theory was tested and refuted by the presence of a normal arginine vasopressin response, indicating the afferent limb of the carotid sinus reflex is intact.[16] Alternatively, it has been postulated that CSH is due to an abnormality within the central nervous system, specifically upregulation of brainstem postsynaptic alpha-2 adrenoceptors.[17] Carotid sinus stimulation may then cause an exaggerated efferent response, resulting in hypotension and bradycardia. Parry and colleagues[18] embarked on the first attempt to try to prove this theoretical hypothesis by the administration of the central alpha-2 adrenoceptor antagonist yohimbine to 18 older patients with CSH. In this sample of patients, there was no attenuation of the carotid baroreflex, suggesting that this hypothesis needs further elucidation. Another group studying the pathophysiology of the carotid sinus baroreflex observed a high proportion of abnormal sternocleidomastoid electromyographic results in subjects with CSH compared with healthy controls. They offer an explanation of chronic terminal denervation of the sternocleidomastoid muscle by an as yet unknown process causing increased sensitivity of the baroreflex arc. However, a direct cause-and-effect relationship has not been effectively established.[19,20]

Emerging pathologic data in patients with CSH are consistent with a neurodegenerative process in medullary nucleii, which may in turn be associated with impaired baroreceptor regulation.[21] Recent data on heart rate variability and baroreflex sensitivity suggest higher resting sympathetic activity and increased baroreceptor sensitivity in CSH in both symptomatic and asymptomatic subjects. The authors suggest this finding of autonomic dysregulation may be indicative of a generalized autonomic disorder.[22] It is hoped that further research in this area will annotate the pathophysiology of this complex condition.

CLINICAL PRESENTATION AND DIAGNOSIS
Symptoms

The most common symptoms attributed to CSH are dizziness (presyncope) and syncope. Case reports throughout the literature describe typical provocation maneuvers such as head turning, shaving, or the wearing of tight neck collars.[5–7] The onset of symptoms tends to be sudden, of short duration, and with quick recovery. Symptoms may be of longer duration when significant hypotension occurs.[23] Significant injuries, including fractures, are not uncommon due to minimal premonitory symptoms.[24]

Syncope and Falls Overlap

Kenny was the first to hypothesize the overlap between syncope and falls in older patients with unexplained falls.[25] A fall is generally defined as coming to rest on the ground or other lower level without loss of consciousness. Seven patients with recurrent falls who denied associated loss of consciousness underwent carotid sinus massage. A cardioinhibitory response of less than 3 seconds was induced in all patients, and 5 patients had loss of consciousness in the upright position, which they subsequently denied when questioned after recovery. Successive studies by the same investigators have yielded similar findings.[26] Richardson and colleagues[27] performed carotid sinus massage in 279 patients over the age of 50 years who presented to emergency with unexplained or recurrent falls. A total of 34% of fallers had a positive response: 23% cardioinhibitory and 11% vasodepressor. The previously described amnesia for loss of consciousness may explain the overlap between syncope and falls. An accurate history of falling is often difficult to obtain due to poor recall, even in independently living, cognitively intact older persons.[28] Also, a witness account is frequently unavailable.[26]

Diagnosis

Carotid sinus syndrome (CSS) is diagnosed when a hypersensitive response to carotid massage is produced in patients presenting with syncope or other symptoms (as previously described). A cardioinhibitory response is referred to as cardioinhibitory CSS (CICSS), and a vasodepressor response is vasodepressor CSS (VDCSS). CSS is widely accepted as a condition related to aging, as it is rarely identified in patients under the age of 50 years.[29] There is differing opinion whether reproduction of spontaneous symptoms in association with a hypersensitive response is required for the diagnosis.[30]

Carotid Sinus Massage

The technique for stimulating the carotid sinus has fluctuated over the past century. In 1932, digital pressure applied to the carotid sinus for 10 to 20 seconds with the patient in a supine position was the method described.[31] Weiss and Baker detailed a similar technique but included the observation that symptoms were more readily induced in the upright position.[7] Subsequently, Lown and Levine described the technique of 5 seconds of gentle massage.[32] Around the same time, Franke published a method of stimulation for 10 to 30 seconds, terminated if asystole of 2 to 3 seconds was induced.[11] Thomas adapted Franke's technique, starting with 20 seconds of gentle massage followed by 15 seconds of longitudinal massage, using pressure insufficient to occlude the ipsilateral temporal arterial pulse. If a response was not elicited, the test was repeated in the supine position.[33]

By the 1980s, the general consensus was that external stimulation of the carotid sinus should be by longitudinal massage; the force applied should not occlude the carotid artery, and the duration should not exceed 5 seconds.[34] Clearly, this procedure has inherent difficulties relating to both the patient and the clinician that make standardization challenging.

The European Society of Cardiology guidelines detail the currently accepted protocols for CSM.[35] The procedure should be done with the patient in both the supine and upright positions. Continuous electrocardiographic monitoring and noninvasive blood pressure monitoring are recommended. Following baseline measurements, carotid massage is performed for 5 to 10 seconds at the anterior margin of the sternocleidomastoid muscle at the level of the cricoid cartilage (**Box 4**). If a positive result is not obtained, the procedure is then repeated on the opposite side after an interval of 1 to 2 minutes. The importance

---

Box 4
Carotid sinus massage

- CSM is performed for 5 to 10 seconds.
- One-third of patients have a positive response only in the upright position.
- Continuous heart rate monitoring and blood pressure monitoring during CSM are preferable.

---

of performing the procedure in the upright position is increasingly recognized, as one-third of patients will only have a positive response in the upright position.[36,37] If a cardioinhibitory response is elicited, atropine may be administered before repeating massage to determine the degree of contributory vasodepression. Determining the contribution of vasodepression to symptoms is clinically relevant, as pacemaker therapy may be less effective in the mixed form as opposed to the cardioinhibitory type.[24,38]

Complications of CSM

Complications attributed to CSM can be divided into 2 categories: neurologic and cardiovascular (**Box 5**). The bulk of reported data comes from a single center, Newcastle upon Tyne, United Kingdom. Davies and colleagues[39] reported on 4000 patients who underwent testing in the supine and upright positions and on both right and left sides, for a total of 16,000 episodes of CSM. Eleven patients had neurologic complications associated with the procedure, half occurring within 5 minutes and the rest within 2 hours. In 82% of patients (9 patients), symptoms resolved completely by 1 month. There were no cardiovascular complications. The same center prospectively collected data on 1000 consecutive patients with syncope or unexplained falls who underwent 3805 episodes of carotid massage.

Box 5
Complications of CSM

- Neurologic and cardiovascular complications have been reported during CSM.
- Cardiovascular complications (primarily arrhythmia) are extremely rare.
- Transient neurologic symptoms and signs occur in up to 0.9% of patients.
- Persistent neurologic deficits are extremely rare following CSM.
- CSM should be considered a safe, low-risk procedure.

Neurologic complications were defined as any abnormal sensations or visual symptoms, paraesthesia, paresis, or cognitive dysfunction. Nine patients reported symptoms or signs consistent with a neurologic complication, all immediately following discontinuation of carotid massage. Complete resolution occurred within 10 minutes in 7 patients. Of the remaining 2 patients, 1 experienced recovery within 24 hours, but the other was left with a residual deficit of the right hand. Cardiovascular complications did not occur.[40] Other groups have reported similarly low complication rates.[30,41]

In summary, neurologic complications related to CSM are rare and persisting deficits even rarer, with a rate of approximately 1 case in 1000 patients. There are no clinical predictors for these complications. Adverse cardiovascular effects are largely confined to the occasional case report.[42,43] CSM should be considered a safe, low-risk procedure.

Overlap with Vasovagal Syncope

Kenny and colleagues[25] reported the attributable diagnosis in 65 consecutive older patients undergoing standardized investigation in a syncope clinic over a 6-month period. Of the 26 patients diagnosed with VDCSH, 5 also met diagnostic criteria for vasovagal syncope, suggesting the possibility of a common etiology.[24] Alboni and colleagues[44] also concluded that there was much overlap in the clinical spectrum of neurally mediated reflex syncope, including CSH and vasovagal syncope. However, a recent large retrospective case-control study failed to show a similar overlap; vasovagal syncope was common in patients with CSH, but was also prevalent in patients without CSH. Rather than a similar mechanism, the authors concluded that the overlap was more likely due to the coexistence of common conditions in older patients.[45]

EPIDEMIOLOGY

The prevalence of CSH in the literature is variable, dependent upon method, definition of a hypersensitive response, and the patient population studied. There are several published case series of heart rate and blood pressure response to carotid sinus massage. Parry[1] originally studied those with a diagnosis of angina; subsequent reports also found a high incidence in the presence of ischemic and/or structural heart disease.[7,10,46] More recently, 118 consecutive patients with chest pain and coronary artery disease underwent CSM before coronary angiography. Forty patients (26.6%) had CSH, the prevalence highest among those with multivessel disease,[47] leading to the postulation that atherosclerosis is an etiologic factor in the development of CSH.

The most frequently studied group is composed of older patients with unexplained syncope. Kumar and colleagues[48] performed CSM on 265 subjects over 60 years of age, 130 of whom had syncope of unknown cause. Twenty-nine patients (22.3%) had an abnormal response, resulting in a diagnosis of CSS. There was no significant difference in the proportion of vasodepressor or cardioinhibitory responses. Consistent with other publications, there was a preponderance of men in the positive group with a rate approximately four times that in women. Volkmann and colleagues[49] investigated 210 patients (108 men, mean age 61.1 ± 28.1 years) with syncope or dizziness, and 87 patients (41%) demonstrated cardioinhibition with asystole of at least 3 seconds. One hundred patients with recurrent unexplained syncope despite a standardized evaluation had carotid sinus massage performed in both the supine and upright positions. Their mean age was 60 ± 18 years, and 54 were men. Forty nine per cent of patients demonstrated either a cardioinhibitory (39%) or vasodepressor response (10%), with reproduction of syncope during CSM in 37 patients.[50]

In summary, the prevalence of CSH in patients with unexplained syncope ranges from 22.3% to 68% and is likely dependent upon a number of factors including patient characteristics (ie, age and gender), technique used to provoke a hypersensitive response (5 vs 10 seconds of CSM, supine vs upright patient positioning), operator experience, and definition of a positive result (**Box 6**).[48–51]

Several investigators have studied the response to CSM in asymptomatic older individuals, demonstrating a hypersensitive response in 0% to 20% of this population.[48–51] In 25 healthy older persons (61–87 years), 3 people (12%) had a vasodepressor response of greater than 50 mm Hg, and no one had a cardioinhibitory response.[52] Another series of 95 healthy older individuals aged over 65

(mean 74) years who underwent CSM had a positive result in 4.2% of subjects.[53]

The largest series to date of an unselected population of community-dwelling older persons was published by Kenny's group.[54] A total of 272 individuals underwent carotid sinus massage in both the supine and upright position; a subgroup of 80 persons had not previously experienced symptoms of dizziness, syncope, or unexplained falls. The baseline clinical characteristics of the subgroup did not differ significantly from the total group. CSH was identified in 28 of 80 (35%) of those without prior symptoms.

In summary, CSH is present in up to 68% of older patients with previously undiagnosed syncope and in up to 35% of asymptomatic community-dwelling persons aged over 65 years. Although it is generally accepted that interventions such as pacing for cardioinhibition reduces symptoms, more recent data question the causal effect between CSH and syncope (and/or falls), suggesting that CSH may merely be an age-related clinical finding with no relation to symptoms.

PROGNOSIS

The natural history of CSH and CSS is not well established (**Box 7**). One prospective study of 60 patients with CSS who were randomized to permanent pacing versus no pacing reported symptom recurrence in 57% of those in the pacing group compared with only 9% in those in the no pacing group.[55] The same group followed 262 patients with symptoms of presyncope or syncope due to CSH, as well as 55 patients with unexplained syncope, over a mean time of 44 plus or minus 24 months. There was no reported difference in mortality between the 2 groups. Furthermore, the mortality rate was similar to that of the general population.[56] Huang and colleagues[57] performed electrophysiological studies and CSM in 76 patients with unexplained syncope. Twenty-one patients (28%) had CICSH. Of these, 13 patients selectively underwent permanent pacemaker implantation, based on symptom reproduction during CSM, evidence of sinoatrial and/or atrioventricular node disease, or presence of coronary artery disease.

Box 6
Epidemiology of CSH

- CSH is common in patients with hypertension and coronary artery disease.
- In unexplained syncope, the prevalence of CSH ranges from 22% to 68%.
- There is an overlap between symptoms of syncope and falls.
- CSH is present in up to 35% of asymptomatic older persons.

Box 7
Prognosis

- The prognosis of CSS is not well established.
- Patients left untreated will usually have recurrent symptoms.
- The natural history of asymptomatic patients with CSH is unknown.

There was no recurrence of syncope in the pacing group patients in 42 ± 19 months of follow-up. One of the 8 patients not in the pacing group had syncope during follow-up. Another series of 65 consecutive older patients with syncope and/or unexplained falls who were referred to a specialty unit were systematically investigated. Five patients with a cardioinhibitory response to CSM received permanent pacing. During a 6-month follow-up, symptoms were reduced.[26]

In summary, long-term follow-up data mostly consist of observational or selected treatment versus no treatment studies in patients with CSS. Despite these limitations, it is generally accepted that patients with symptoms associated with a hypersensitive response to CSM have a high rate of symptom recurrence. Of note, the natural history and prognosis of symptomatic subjects with a hypersensitive response to carotid massage are not known.

TREATMENT

The treatment of CSH depends on a number of factors, including the hemodynamic response to carotid massage and the patient's clinical history. If there are obvious causative factors such as vigorous head turning or tight shirt collars, these maneuvers/clothing should be minimized and/or avoided. There are scanty randomized trial data to guide the treatment of VDCSS, and therefore no established therapy for this diagnosis. Although there are conflicting trial data, the accepted treatment for CICSS is permanent pacing.

Pharmacologic Treatment

The management of VDCSS is challenging and generally unrewarding. Almquist and colleagues[58] studied the hemodynamic effects of various pharmacologic agents in patients with permanent pacemakers in situ for CICSS and a persistent vasodepressor response to CSM. Atropine and propranolol did not prevent a vasodepressor response. Norepinephrine infusion significantly diminished the vasodepressor response without producing a marked hypertensive response. Similarly, ephedrine attenuated the hypotensive response. However, the sympathomimetic adverse effects are potentially hazardous, particularly in this predominantly older patient population with a high rate of systolic hypertension and coronary artery disease, making these agents unsuitable for clinical use (**Box 8**). Isoproterenol and amphetamines are not efficacious and frequently are poorly tolerated.

There is 1 nonrandomized, uncontrolled report of the use of fludrocortisone in 11 patients with

---

Box 8
Pharmacologic treatment

- Sympathomimetic drugs are potentially harmful and not efficacious.
- There are case reports of successful treatment with SSRIs and fludrocortisone.
- There is only 1 randomized drug trial, showing potentially improved symptoms with midodrine.
- Additional pharmacologic trials are required.

VDCSS.[59] Patients were given 100 µg of fludrocortisone and underwent repeat CSM 2 weeks later. There was a significant reduction in the degree of vasodepression compared with baseline: 56 mm Hg versus 32 mm Hg, $P<.01$. Patients also reported less symptoms of presyncope and syncope. Grubb and colleagues,[60] reported 2 patients with CICSS who experienced recurrent syncope despite pacing, due to vasodepression. Both patients were given a serotonin reuptake inhibitor (SSRI) and had complete resolution of symptoms in the short term.

Lastly, a double-blind, randomized placebo-controlled crossover trial of midodrine in 10 older adults with a history of unexplained syncope and an asymptomatic decrease in systolic blood pressure of greater than 50 mm Hg or a symptomatic decrease of greater than 30 mm Hg within 30 seconds of CSM was reported.[61] Midodrine significantly reduced both the rate of symptom reporting and the degree of vasodepression during CSM. It also increased the mean 24-h ambulatory blood pressure compared with baseline, 133/75 mm Hg versus 127/70 mm Hg, which may limit its clinical usefulness.

Permanent Pacing

The first published report of using a permanent pacemaker to treat CSH was by Voss in 1970 (**Box 9**).[62] He described the case of an 81-year-old woman with a 4-year history of recurrent syncope. During CSM, a 3.5 second period of asystole associated with syncope occurred. A single-chamber (VVI) pacemaker was inserted followed by repeat CSM, showing slowing of the ventricular rate, interrupted after 1000 milliseconds by ventricular pacing, in the absence of symptoms. The authors acknowledge that although the patient remained asymptomatic, the follow-up was brief.

A case series of 10 patients was reported in 1973.[63] Inclusion criteria were a clinical history of syncope, a positive response to CSM (defined as asystole or marked bradycadia), and syncope during massage. All patients had a VVI pacemaker inserted, and all remained symptom free during follow-up, which ranged from 6 to 55 months. A decade later, Morley and colleagues[64] published a series of 70 patients who underwent permanent pacing for CICSH following extensive clinical and electrophysiological assessment. The criteria for permanent pacing included reproduction of symptomatic asystole greater than 3 seconds and abolition of symptoms by temporary ventricular pacing during repeated CSM. The presenting symptom in 61 patients was syncope, and 9 patients described severe presyncope. During a mean follow-up of 18 months, 77%[54] of patients experienced complete resolution of symptoms. Of the remaining 16 patients with persistent symptoms, 8 had atrial pacing, atrial sensing, inhibit (AAI) pacemakers. During CSM, symptomatic atrioventricular block occurred in all 8 patients; changing to either dual-chamber or ventricular-based pacing abolished symptoms. A series of 89 patients with CICSS who had permanent pacemakers inserted and were followed for up to 17 years reported no syncope recurrence.[65] Further observational studies comparing pacing with no pacing have demonstrated a marked reduction in syncope.[57,66] These observational nonrandomized, noncontrolled case series consistently demonstrate almost complete resolution of patient symptoms, predominantly syncope, with permanent pacing. However, due to the aforementioned study design limitations, subsequent randomized trials are warranted to systematically assess the effect of permanent pacing on symptoms.

In 2 randomized trials of pacing versus no pacing, there was less syncope recurrence in paced patients. The first trial included 60 patients with syncope or severe presyncope who experienced reproduction of spontaneous symptoms during CSM associated with ventricular asystole lasting at least 3 seconds. Twenty-eight patients were randomized to no treatment, while 32 patients received permanent pacing. Three (9%) of paced patients had symptom recurrence compared with 16 (57%) patients in the no pacing group during 36 plus or minus 10 months of follow-up.[55] Claesson and colleagues[67] subsequently randomized 60 patients with a history of syncope, ventricular aystole of at least 3 seconds in response to CSS, and an otherwise negative work-up for syncope, to either pacing or no pacing. The rate of syncope recurrence in the 12-month follow-up period in the pacing group was 10% compared with 40% in the no pacing group (*P* = .008). The majority of the syncope recurrences in the no pacing group occurred during the first 3 months of follow-up (11 of 12 patients). Although these 2 studies were designed in a randomized fashion, there was no blinding of treatment to address the placebo effect of a significant procedural intervention.

Until 2001, pacing trials for CICSS only included patients with either severe presyncope or syncope. Kenny and colleagues[68] then reported a randomized controlled trial of dual-chamber cardiac pacing versus no pacing in 175 patients over 50 years of age presenting to emergency departments with a nonaccidental fall and cardioinhibitory CSH. Those patients who received a pacemaker had a significant reduction in their mean number of falls, from 9.3 to 4.1 falls in the 1year follow-up period. Interestingly, the number of patients who fell was similar in the intervention and control groups. This trial was not blinded and therefore does not address the potential placebo effect in the treatment group. The same group subsequently reported 2 further randomized trials in patients with unexplained falls and a cardioinhibitory response to CSM. The first, a randomized double-blind crossover trial, included 34 patients over the age of 55 years.[69] All patients received a dual-chamber permanent pacemaker, which was turned on (DDD mode) or off (ODO mode) for 6 months, then crossed over to the alternate mode for a further 6 months. Pacing (DDD mode) had no effect on the number of falls or the percentage of patients who fell. The authors noted there was a reduction in the number of falls in both 6-month periods compared with the number of falls in the 6 months before enrollment, suggesting the potential for a placebo effect of pacing. The Syncope and Falls in the Elderly: Pacing and Carotid Sinus Evaluation (SAFE

PACE) 2 trial, an international multicenter randomized controlled trial of permanent pacing in unexplained fallers with CICSH, included 141 patients from 22 centers.[70] Patients were randomized to either dual-chamber pacing or an implantable loop recorder (ILR), in an attempt to address the potential placebo effect, and followed for 24 months. No significant reduction in falls was seen between the paced patients and those who received ILRs.

In summary, despite a paucity of randomized controlled trials, permanent pacing has become established treatment for CICSH during the past 40 years.[71] Small observational nonrandomized noncontrolled studies support pacing in patients with syncope or presyncope that is reproduced during CSM-induced asystole.[30] Randomized controlled trials in patients with unexplained falls have shown conflicting results, suggesting further research is required to determine if pacing is effective. Most published studies do not adequately address the powerful placebo effect of permanent pacing.

Pacing Mode

The choice of pacing mode between dual-chamber pacing and ventricular-based pacing is debatable. Of note, single-chamber atrial-based pacing is not appropriate for CSS due to the high rate of atrioventricular node (AV) block in these patients.[64] A randomized controlled trial of DDI versus VVI pacing in elderly syncopal patients with CICSH supported a reduction in symptoms with dual-chamber pacing.[72] Similarly, data from Brignole and colleagues[38,73] substantiated a preference for dual-chamber pacing, with less symptomatic hypotension. Current guidelines state that dual-chamber pacing is generally preferred over single-chamber pacing.[74] More recently, however, a double-blind crossover trial comparing dual pacing (atrium and ventricle), dual sensing (atrium and ventricle), dual (inhibit and trigger), rate-responsive (DDDR), DDDR with sudden bradycardia response, or VVI pacing did not show a significant reduction in symptoms between the 3 modes of pacing.[75]

Carotid Sinus Denervation

Carotid sinus denervation either by radiation or surgery has been propounded as a treatment modality for more than 60 years (**Box 10**).[76,77] Neither method has been rigorously applied in a clinical trial and has the potential to harm.[78] The 2 largest surgical case series reported include 19 and 8 patients, followed for 15 years and 30 months, respectively.[79,80] The procedure appears

---

Box 10
Carotid sinus denervation

- Carotid sinus denervation, either surgically or with radiation therapy, has been reported.
- A reduction in symptoms and minimal complications during long-term follow-up have been reported.
- There are no clinical trial data to support carotid sinus denervation.
- This treatment is rarely used now.

---

to afford long-term symptom relief with minimal complications in selected centers. However, this form of treatment has largely been abandoned over the past 2 decades.

SUMMARY

CSH was first reported more than 200 years ago. Nevertheless, the complete understanding of this relatively common clinical finding in older patients has proven elusive. There is evidence to support an association between symptoms, particularly syncope, and a hypersensitive response to CSM. However, the clinical implications of a high prevalence in asymptomatic healthy older persons is not known. A central degenerative process likely underlies the pathophysiology, but this is, as yet, unproven. Although selected patients have had symptom improvement with treatment, particularly with permanent pacing, there is a dearth of randomized controlled trial data to guide management.

REFERENCES

1. Parry CH. An inquiry into the symptoms and causes of the syncope anginosa commonly called angina pectoris. London: Bath; 1799.
2. Krediet CT, Parry SW, Jardine DL, et al. The history of diagnosing carotid sinus hypersensitivity: why are the current criteria too sensitive? Europace 2011;13:14–22.
3. Hering HE. Der Sinus caroticus an der Ursprungsstelle der Carotis interna als Ausgangsort eines hemmenden Herzreflexes und depressorischen Gefässreflexes. MMW Munch Med Wochenschr 1924;71:701–5.
4. Sigler LH. Clinical observations on the carotid sinus reflex: I the frequency and the degree of response to carotid sinus pressure under various diseased states. Am J Med Sci 1933;186:110–8.
5. Roskam J. Un syndrome nouveau. Syncopes cardiaques graves et syncopes repetees par hyperreflexivite sinocarotidienne. Presse Med 1930;38:590–1.

6. Nathanson MH. Hyperactive cardioinhibitory carotid sinus reflex. Arch Intern Med 1946;77:491–503.

7. Weiss S, Baker JP. The carotid sinus reflex in health and disease: its role in the causation of fainting and convulsions. Medicine. Wien Arch f inn Med 1933; 12:297–354.

8. Brignole M, Alboni P, Benditt DG, et al. Guidelines on management (diagnosis and treatment) of syncope—update 2004: executive summary. Eur Heart J 2004;25:2054–72.

9. Brignole M, Alboni P, Benditt DG, et al. Guideline on management (diagnosis and treatment) of syncope. Eur Heart J 2001;22:1256–306.

10. Sigler LH. Hyperactive cardioinhibitory carotid sinus reflex. Arch Intern Med 1941;67:177.

11. Franke H. On the hyperactive carotid sinus syndrome. Acta Neuroveg (Wien) 1963;25:187–203.

12. Luck JC, Hoover RJ, Biederman RW, et al. Observations on carotid sinus hypersensitivity from direct intraneural recordings of sympathetic nerve traffic. Am J Cardiol 1996;77:1362.

13. Hainsworth R. Clinical guide to cardiac autonomic tests. In: Malik M, editor. Physiology of the cardiac autonomic system. Dordrecht (The Netherlands): Kluwer Academic Publishers; 1998. p. 3–28.

14. Herbert H, Moga MM, Saper CB. Connections of the parabrachial nucleus with the nucleus of the solitary tract and the medullary reticular formation in the rat. J Comp Neurol 1990;4(293):540–80.

15. Chapleau MW, Abboud FM. Cardiovascular reflex control in health and disease. In: Hainsworth R, Mark AL, editors. Mechanisms of adaption and resetting of the baroreceptor reflex. London: Saunders; 1993. p. 165–94.

16. Kenny RA, Lyon CC, Ingram AM, et al. Enhanced vagal activity and normal arginine vasopressin response in carotid sinus syndrome: implications for a central abnormality in carotid sinus hypersensitivity. Cardiovasc Res 1987;21:45–50.

17. O'Mahony D. Pathophysiology of carotid sinus hypersensitivity in elderly patients. Lancet 1995; 346:950–2.

18. Parry SW, Baptist M, Gilroy JJ, et al. Central ∞2 adrenoceptors and the pathogenesis of carotid sinus hypersensitivity. Heart 2004;90:935–6.

19. Tea SH, Mansourati J, L'Heveder G, et al. New insights into the pathophysiology of carotid sinus syndrome. Circulation 1996;93(7):1411–6.

20. Blanc JJ, L'Heveder G, Mansourati J, et al. Assessment of a newly recognized association: carotid sinus hypersensitivity and denervation of sternocleidomastoid muscles. Circulation 1997;95:2548–51.

21. Miller VM, Kenny RA, Slade JY, et al. Medullary autonomic pathology in carotid sinus hypersensitivity. Neuropathol Appl Neurobiol 2008;34:403–11.

22. Tan MP, Kenny RA, Chadwick TJ, et al. Carotid sinus hypersensitivity: disease state or clinical sign of ageing? Insights from a controlled study of autonomic function in symptomatic and asymptomatic subjects. Europace 2010;12:1630–6.

23. Wieling W, Thijs RD, van Dijk N, et al. Symptoms and signs of syncope: a review of the link between physiology and clinical clues. Brain 2009;132:2630–42.

24. McIntosh SJ, Lawson J, Kenny RA. Clinical characteristics of vasodepressor, cardioinhibitory and mixed carotid sinus syndrome in the elderly. Am J Med 1993;95:203–8.

25. Kenny RA, Traynor G. Carotid sinus syndrome—clinical characteristics in elderly patients. Age Ageing 1991;20:449–54.

26. McIntosh S, Da Costa D, Kenny RA. Outcome of an integrated approach to the investigation of dizziness, falls and syncope in elderly patients referred to a 'syncope' clinic. Age Ageing 1993;22:53–8.

27. Richardson DA, Bexton RS, Shaw FE. Prevalence of cardioinhibitory carotid sinus hypersensitivity in patients 50 years or over presenting to the accident and emergence department with "unexplained" or "recurrent" falls. Pacing Clin Electrophysiol 1997; 20:820–3.

28. Cummings SR, Nevitt MC, Kidd S. Forgetting falls: the limited accuracy of recall of falls in the elderly. J Am Geriatr Soc 1988;36:613–6.

29. Humm AM, Mathias CJ. Unexplained syncope—is screening for carotid sinus hypersensitivity indicated in all patients aged >40 years? J Neurol Neurosurg Psychiatr 2006;77:1267–70.

30. Puggioni E, Guiducci V, Brignole M, et al. Results and complications of carotid sinus massage performed according to the 'method of symptoms.' Am J Cardiol 2002;89:599–601.

31. Mandelstamm M, Lifschitz S. Die Wirkung der Karotissinusreflexe auf den Blutdruck beim Menschen. Wien Arch F inn Med 1932;22:397.

32. Lown B, Levine SA. The carotid sinus—clinical value. Circulation 1961;23:766.

33. Thomas JE. Hyperactive carotid sinus reflex and carotid sinus syncope. Mayo Clin Proc 1969;44: 127–39.

34. Morley CA, Sutton R. Carotid sinus syncope. Int J Cardiol 1984;6:287–93.

35. The Task Force on Syncope. Guidelines on management (diagnosis and treatment) of syncope—update. Europace 2004;6:467–537.

36. Brignole M, Sartore B, Prato R. Role of body position during carotid sinus stimulation test in the diagnosis of cardioinhibitory carotid sinus syndrome. G Ital Cardiol 1983;14:69–72.

37. Parry SW, Richardson D, O'Shea D, et al. Diagnosis of carotid sinus hypersensitivity in older adults: carotid sinus massage in the upright position is essential. Heart 2000;83:22–3.

38. Brignole M, Menozzi C, Lolli G, et al. Validation of a method for choice of pacing mode in carotid sinus

syndrome with or without sinus bradycardia. Pacing Clin Electrophysiol 1991;14:196–203.

39. Davies AJ, Kenny RA. Frequency of neurologic complications following carotid sinus massage. Am J Cardiol 1998;81(10):1256–7.

40. Richardson DA, Bexton R, Shaw FE, et al. Complications of carotid sinus massage—a prospective series of older patients. Age Ageing 2000;29:413–7.

41. Walsh T, Clinch D, Cosetelloe A, et al. Carotid sinus massage—how safe is it? Age Ageing 2006;35:518–20.

42. Matthews OA. Ventricular tachycardia induced by carotid sinus stimulation. J Maine Med Assoc 1969;60:135–6.

43. Alexander S, Ping WC. Fatal ventricular fibrillation during carotid sinus stimulation. Am J Cardiol 1966;18:289–91.

44. Alboni P, Brignole M, Menozzi C, et al. Clinical spectrum of neurally mediated reflex syncope. Europace 2004;6:55–62.

45. Tan MP, Newton JL, Chadwick TJ, et al. The relationship between carotid sinus hypersenstivity, orthostatic hypotension, and vasovagal syncope: a case-control study. Europace 2008;10:1400–5.

46. Smiddy J, Lewis HD, Dunn M. The effect of carotid massage in older men. J Gerontol 1972;27:209.

47. Tsioufis CP, Kallikazaros IE, Toutouzas KP, et al. Exaggerated carotid sinus massage responses are related to severe coronary artery disease in patients being evaluated for chest pain. Clin Cardiol 2002;25:161–6.

48. Kumar NP, Thomas A, Mudd P, et al. The usefulness of carotid sinus massage in different patient groups. Age Ageing 2003;32:666–9.

49. Volkmann H, Schnerch B, Kuhnert H. Diagnostic value of carotid sinus hypersensitivity. PACE 1990;13:2065–70.

50. Brignole M, Menozzi C, Gianfranchi L. Carotid sinus massage, eyeball compression, and head-up tilt test in patients with syncope of uncertain origin and in health control subjects. Am Heart J 1991;122:1644–51.

51. Morillo CA, Camacho ME, Wood MA, et al. Diagnostic utility of mechanical, pharmacological and orthostatic stimulation of the carotid sinus in patients with unexplained syncope. J Am Coll Cardiol 1999;34:1587–94.

52. McIntosh S, Lawson J, Kenny RA. Heart rate blood pressure responses to carotid sinus massage in healthy elderly subjects. Age Ageing 1994;23:57–61.

53. Jeffreys M, Wood DA, Lampe F. The heart rate response to carotid artery massage in a sample of healthy elderly people. Pacing Clin Electrophysiol 1996;19:1488–92.

54. Kerr SJ, Pearce MS, Brayne C, et al. Carotid sinus hypersensitivity in asymptomatic older persons. Arch Intern Med 2006;166:515–20.

55. Brignole M, Menozzi C, Lolli G, et al. Long-term outcome of paced and no-paced patients with severe carotid sinus syndrome. Am J Cardiol 1992;69:1039–43.

56. Brignole M, Oddone D, Cogorno S, et al. Long-term outcome in symptomatic carotid sinus hypersensitivity. Am Heart J 1992;123:687–92.

57. Huang S, Ezri MD, Hauser RG, et al. Carotid sinus hypersensitivity in patients with unexplained syncope: clinical, electrophysiological and long-term follow-up observations. Age Ageing 1988;116(4):989–96.

58. Almquist A, Gornick C, Benson W. Carotid sinus hypersensitivity: evaluation of the vasodepressor component. Circulation 1985;71(5):927–36.

59. DaCosta D, McIntosh S, Kenny RA. Benefits of fludrocortisone in the treatment of symptomatic vasodepressor carotid sinus syndrome. Br Heart J 1993;69:308–10.

60. Grubb BP, Samoil D, Kosinski D, et al. The use of serotonin reuptake inhibitors for the treatment of recurrent syncope due to carotid sinus hypersensitivity unresponsive to dual chamber cardiac pacing. Pacing Clin Electrophysiol 1994;17:1434–6.

61. Moore A, Watts M, Sheehy T, et al. Treatment of vasodepressor carotid sinus syndrome with midodrine: a randomized, controlled pilot study. J Am Geriatr Soc 2005;53:114–8.

62. Voss DM, Magnin GE. Demand pacing and carotid sinus syncope. Am Heart J 1970;79:544–7.

63. Peretz DI, Gerein AN, Miyagishima RT. Permanent demand pacing for hypersensitive carotid sinus syndrome. Can Med Assoc J 1973;108:1131–4.

64. Morley CA, Perrins EJ, Grant P, et al. Carotid sinus syncope treated by pacing. Analysis of persistent symptoms and role of atrioventricular sequential pacing. Br Heart J 1982;47:411–8.

65. Peretz DI, Abdulla A. Management of cardioinhibitory hypersensitive carotid sinus syncope with permanent cardiac pacing – a seventeen year prospective study. Can J Cardiol 1985;1(2):86–91.

66. Sugrue DD, Gersh BJ, Holmes DR, et al. Symptomatic "isolated" carotid sinus hypersensitivity: natural history and results of treatment with anticholinergic drugs or pacemaker. J Am Coll Cardiol 1986;7(1):158–62.

67. Claesson JE, Kristensson BE, Edvardsson N, et al. Less syncope and milder symptoms in patients treated with pacing for induced cardioinhibitory carotid sinus syndrome: a randomized study. Europace 2007;9:932–6.

68. Kenny RA, Richardson DA, Steen N, et al. Carotid sinus syndrome: a modifiable risk factor for nonaccidental falls in older adults (SAFE PACE). J Am Coll Cardiol 2001;38:1491–6.

69. Parry SW, Steen N, Bexton RS, et al. Pacing in elderly recurrent fallers with carotid sinus

hypersensitivity: a randomised, double-blind, placebo controlled crossover trial. Heart 2009;95: 405–9.

70. Ryan DJ, Steen N, Seifer CM, et al. Carotid sinus syndrome, should we pace? A multicentre, randomised control trial (SAFEPACE 2). Heart 2012; 96:347–51.

71. Epstein AE, DiMarco JP, Ellenbogen KA, et al. ACC/ AHA/HRS 2008 guidelines for device-based therapy of cardiac rhythm abnormalities: a report of the American College of Cardiology/American Heart Association Task Force on Practice Guidelines (Writing Committee to Revise the ACC/AHA/NASPE 2002 Guideline Update for Implantation of Cardiac Pacemakers and Antiarrhythmia Devices). J Am Coll Cardiol 2008;51:e1–62.

72. McIntosh SJ, Lawson J, Bexton RS, et al. A study comparing VVI and DDI pacing in elderly patients with carotid sinus syndrome. Heart 1997; 77:553–7.

73. Brignole M, Sartore B, Barra M, et al. Is DDD superior to VVI pacing in mixed carotid sinus syndrome? An acute and medium-term study. Pacing Clin Electrophysiol 1988;11:1902–10.

74. The Task Force for the Diagnosis and Management of Syncope of the European Society of Cardiology (ESC). Guidelines for the diagnosis and management of syncope (version 2009). Eur Heart J 2009;30: 2631–731.

75. Mcleod CJ, Trusty JM, Jenkins SM, et al. Method of pacing does not affect the recurrence of syncope in carotid sinus syndrome. Pacing Clin Electrophysiol 2012;35:827–33.

76. Stevenson CA. The role of roentgen therapy in the carotid sinus syndrome. Radiology 1939;32:209.

77. Greeley HP, Smedal MI, Morset W. The treatment of the carotid sinus syndrome by irradiation. N Engl J Med 1955;252:91–4.

78. Ford FR. Fatal hypertensive crisis following denervation of the carotid sinus for relief of repeated attacks of syncope. Bull Johns Hopkins Hosp 1957;100:14–6.

79. Trout HH, Brown LL, Thompson JE. Carotid sinus syndrome: treatment by carotid sinus denervation. Ann Surg 1979;189:575–80.

80. Fachinetti P, Bellochi S, Dorizzi A, et al. Carotid sinus syndrome: a review of the literature and our experience using carotid sinus denervation. J Neurosurg Sci 1998;42:189–93.

Treatment of Neurally Mediated Reflex Syncope

Juan C. Guzman, MD, MSc, FRCPC[a],
Luciana V. Armaganijan, MD[b],
Carlos A. Morillo, MD, FRCPC, FESC, FHRS[a,c],*

KEYWORDS

• Syncope • Vasovagal • Neurally mediated • Pharmacology

KEY POINTS

- Vasovagal syncope (VVS) is the most frequent cause of recurrent syncope.
- VVS has a benign course, but quality of life can be impaired by recurrent episodes of syncope.
- Nonpharmacologic measures are simple and usually safe and should be tried as first-line therapy in patients with frequent syncope and no obvious contraindications.
- Pharmacologic therapy is recommended in patients refractory to nonpharmacologic interventions. No specific guidelines are available to decide which pharmacologic treatment should be initiated; however, midodrine seems to be the most promising agent in practice, and β-blockade may have a role in older patients.

INTRODUCTION

Neurally mediated reflex syncope, more commonly known as vasovagal syncope (VVS), is the most common cause of transient loss of consciousness in adults. It affects at least 20% of individuals at some time in their lives.[1] Despite its benign course, recurrent reflex syncope may be highly symptomatic in about a third of patients, leading to significant deterioration of quality of life with psychological, driving, employment, and financial implications.[1] Several nonpharmacologic therapies have been developed, which include counterpressure maneuvers (CPMs), orthostatic training, and salt and fluid intake. These simple interventions, in addition to counseling and education of patients, are usually successful in reducing the frequency and recurrence of syncope. The initial therapeutic approach should always include counseling and avoidance of potential triggers of VVS. Simple measures, based on scarce evidence, such as increased water and NaCl intake, should be routinely implemented as first-line therapy. Education geared to improving patients' understanding of the early onset of prodromal symptoms is essential to improve response to therapy.

A clear and reproducible prodromal symptom complex is essential for the successful implementation of CPMs. Younger patients tend to have typical prodromal symptoms that are easy to identify and that provide the basis for the successful interventions that can markedly reduce recurrence of syncope. Multiple pharmacologic interventions and electrical therapy with pacemakers have been tested in small trials, with conflicting results. This article reviews the bulk of evidence available on the different types of therapeutic strategies currently available for the management of VVS. The role of pacemakers is reviewed in the by Moya and colleagues elsewhere in this issue.

[a] Department of Medicine, McMaster University, 237 Barton Street East, Hamilton, Ontario L8L 2X2, Canada;
[b] Arrhythmia Service, Dante Pazzanese Institute of Cardiology, Sao Paulo, Brazil Vila Mariana CEP 04012–909;
[c] Cardiology Division, Department of Medicine, Syncope & Autonomic Disorder Unit, David Braley CVSRI, Room C-3-120, 237 Barton Street East, Hamilton, Ontario, Canada
* Corresponding author. Cardiology Division, Department of Medicine, Director Syncope & Autonomic Disorder Unit, David Braley CVSRI, Room C-3-120, 237 Barton Street East, Hamilton, Ontario, Canada.
E-mail addresses: morillo@hhsc.ca; carlos.morillo@phri.ca

Cardiol Clin 31 (2013) 123–129
http://dx.doi.org/10.1016/j.ccl.2012.10.007
0733-8651/13/$ – see front matter © 2013 Elsevier Inc. All rights reserved.

PATHOPHYSIOLOGY OF VVS

An in-depth review of the complex mechanisms that trigger the vasovagal response is beyond the scope of this article, and is reviewed in the article by Jardine elsewhere in this issue. In brief, orthostatic stress in susceptible subjects leads to a myriad of physiologic responses that attempt to restore the homeostatic and physiologic mechanisms that maintain blood pressure when in the upright position. Reduction of venous return in the upright posture triggers increased vagal efferent traffic that in turn leads to increased sympathetic central and peripheral activity.[2] These responses are associated with complex neurohumoral changes that lead in turn to the eventual response of hypotension and bradycardia. These responses reduce cerebral perfusion, causing the transient loss of consciousness.

NONPHARMACOLOGIC INTERVENTIONS

Nonpharmacologic interventions are primarily focused on improving overall volume and reflex response caused by orthostatic stress or other triggers. Nonpharmacologic treatment of VVS is recommended as the first-line therapy and should be instituted in all patients with recurrent VVS.[1] Counseling and education are pillars of treatment and are an integral part of successful treatment of VVS.[1] Treatment of VVS is indicated in patients with recurrent syncope and possibly also in patients with frequent presyncope with the goal of reducing time to first recurrence and overall burden of syncope. In general, these simple interventions are recommended regardless of the frequency of symptoms. Nonpharmacologic interventions are summarized in **Box 1**.

Education and Counseling

Patients seeking medical advice after experiencing an episode of VVS have usually undergone costly diagnostic examinations and are anxious to determine the cause of their syncopal episodes. In this respect, education and counseling provides significant reassurance regarding the benign nature of this condition. Simple descriptions of the physiologic

---

mechanisms that lead to VVS usually reassure the patient, and provide the foundation for the specific interventions.[3] Understanding the typical prodromal symptoms is essential for a successful outcome once the maneuvers are implemented. Identifying and potentially avoiding known triggers (ie, venipuncture, volume depletion, environmental triggers) should be discussed.[4] No randomized controlled trials (RCTs) have systematically assessed any of the reviewed therapeutic strategies; nonetheless, clinical experience suggests that these interventions pose no harm and may improve outcomes and reduce the frequency of episodes.[1,5] Concomitant need of other pharmacologic treatments, such as those used for chronic vasodilator therapy, should be reassessed and adjusted accordingly.[5]

Salt and Water Increase

Volume expansion (ie, increased dietary salt/electrolytes) constitutes one of the cornerstones of treatment of VVS.[1] Plasma volume expansion improves orthostatic tolerance in patients with recurrent VVS.[6–9] Patients should attempt a daily dietary intake of at least 2 g of sodium.[8,9] Urinary sodium excretion may be monitored over 24-hours and 1 or more 1-g salt tablets may be added 3 times a day if needed. The increase in dietary sodium should be accompanied by an increase in fluid intake up to 2 to 2.5 L per day (in adults). Beneficial effects are reported in most subjects within 1 week, particularly in subjects with low dietary salt intake.[10] Patients with known or treated hypertension should not be recommended to increase salt intake.

Rapid water ingestion may prevent VVS recurrence.[3] Previous studies have reported that this intervention is effective in preventing orthostatic intolerance and postprandial hypotension in patients with autonomic failure.[11–14] Moreover, recent reports suggest that water drinking can also be applied to improve orthostatic tolerance in healthy subjects.[15] The rapid onset of the effects of water drinking and its sustained effect support the use of this simple intervention as a preventive measure that can also be used during situations that trigger VVS.[3]

In the absence of contraindications, symptomatic patients should be encouraged to increase their salt and fluid intake to at least 2 g/d of sodium and 2 to 3 L/d of water. Although the evidence supporting this strategy is weak, it is probably a cost-effective and safe strategy that should always be used as first-line therapy.

Orthostatic Training

In highly motivated patients with recurrent VVS, the prescription of progressively prolonged periods of enforced upright posture may reduce syncope

---

> **Box 1**
> **Nonpharmacologic management of VVS**
>
> - Counseling and reassurance (education)
> - Increase in dietary salt intake and water intake
> - Orthostatic training
> - Counterpressure maneuvers

recurrence.[1] Ector and colleagues[16] initially described this technique, in which patients stand with their upper backs positioned against a wall or a corner without moving their arms or legs. Starting at 5 minutes twice daily, over a period of 6 to 8 weeks the tilt training period is gradually increased to as much as 30 to 40 minutes twice daily. The physiologic objective is to reset baroreceptor reflexes, improving gravitational stress response by leading to more efficient vasoconstriction. Orthostatic training can also be achieved by tilt training, and has recently been examined in a group of patients with recurrent VVS.[17] Patients were randomized to treatment with propranolol, disopyramide, or tilt training. On repeat tilt table test, pharmacologic therapy was not effective at preventing syncope (32% propranolol, 26% disopyramide). In contrast, tilt training was highly efficient and prevented syncope in 92% of patients. Di Girolamo and colleagues[18] also studied the efficacy of an orthostatic training program consisting of standing for 40 minutes twice daily. Patients with VVS refractory to standard medical therapy were randomized to a control or orthostatic training group. After a mean follow-up of 18 months, recurrent syncope was experienced by 56.5% in the controlled group, compared with no syncope recurrences in the orthostatic training group. However, low compliance has been reported.[16–19] Three RCTs comparing either orthostatic training or tilt training have failed to confirm reductions in long-term syncope recurrence.[19–21]

In summary, the prescription of progressively prolonged periods of enforced orthostatic training may reduce syncope recurrence in highly motivated young patients when prodromal symptoms are present and reproducible.

Counterpressure Maneuvers

In younger patients, VVS is usually preceded by prodromal symptoms, and appropriate recognition of these provides enough time for CPMs to be implemented. Based on simple physiologic studies, isometric CPMs of the legs (leg crossing) or arms (hand grip and arm tensing) are able to induce a significant blood pressure increase during the phase of impending VVS.[22–24] This effect seems to be mediated largely by sympathetic nerve discharge and vascular resistance increase during maneuvers and by mechanical compression of the venous vascular bed in the legs and abdomen.

Three recent studies have assessed the efficacy and feasibility of CPMs.[22–24] The Physical Counterpressure Maneuvers Trial (PC-Trial)[24] was a multicenter, prospective, randomized clinical trial evaluating the effectiveness of CPMs in 223 patients

(aged 38.6 ± 15.4 years) with recurrent VVS and recognizable prodromal symptoms. Patients were randomly assigned to receive either standardized conventional therapy alone (n = 117) or conventional therapy plus training in CPMs (n = 106). During a mean follow-up period of 14 months, the occurrence of syncope was significantly lower in the group trained in CPMs (50.9% of the patients receiving conventional treatment vs 31.6% of those trained in CPMs; P<.005). Actuarial recurrence-free survival was better in the treatment group, resulting in a significant relative risk reduction of 39% (95% confidence interval [CI], 11%–53%). No adverse events were reported. Other studies have also reported improved quality of life when CPMs are implemented.[25]

In summary, CPMs are effective, feasible, safe, and well accepted by patients in daily life and should be advised as first-line treatment in younger patients presenting with VVS and recognizable prodromal symptoms.

PHARMACOLOGIC TREATMENT

Pharmacologic therapy is usually indicated after nonpharmacologic measures fail to prevent recurrent syncopal episodes. Several agents have been tested with varied results and there is no evidence as to which agent should be started first. **Box 2** lists these agents.

β-Blockers

Based on the initial understanding of the mechanism of VVS, β-blockers were used as first-line therapy. Although early observational studies showed significant reductions in recurrence of syncope, mostly assessed by repeated tilt testing, RCTs have failed to show beneficial effects of β-blockers in unselected patients with recurrent VVS.[26–30]

Metoprolol was proved to be ineffective in preventing syncopal recurrences in the POST,[31] a large multicenter, randomized, placebo-controlled, double-blind study that compared different doses of metoprolol (ranging from 25 to 200 mg daily) to placebo in 208 patients with VVS. No differences in the primary outcome (first recurrence of syncope) were seen between the groups.[31] However, a recent report suggests that, in patients older than 42 years, metoprolol may be effective.[32] Based on a 48% relative risk reduction (RRR) in time to first recurrence of syncope in subjects older than 42 years reported from the POST trial, it is reasonable to try metoprolol in this specific population. An RCT addressing this specific population is being designed.

The latest ESC guidelines[1] do not recommend β-blockers for the routine treatment of

---

Box 2
Pharmacologic agents used to manage VVS

- β-Blockers
  - Not recommended in latest European Society of Cardiology (ESC) guidelines
  - Might be beneficial in patients older than 42 years
- Adrenergic agonists
  - Encouraging results with midodrine recently reported
- Fludrocortisone
  - Available evidence does not show significant reduction in syncope recurrence with fludrocortisone in unselected patients with VVS
  - Further analysis of the Prevention of Syncope Trial (POST) II date may identify subgroups that benefit
- Selective serotonin reuptake inhibitors (SSRIs)
  - Symptomatic patients in whom standard therapies were ineffective, poorly tolerated, or contraindicated are frequently prescribed SSRIs
  - SSRIs may be particularly useful in patients with associated anxiety and panic disorders

---

recurrent VVS; nonetheless, β-blockers are frequently prescribed in VVS and might be beneficial in patients older than 42 years.

α-Agonists

Adrenergic agonists are potent vasoconstrictors that ameliorate the reduction in peripheral resistance responsible for venous pooling and vasodepression, and therefore result in an increase in standing, sitting, and supine systolic and diastolic blood pressure in patients with orthostatic hypotension. Encouraging results with a specific α1-agonist (midodrine) have recently been reported.

Etilefrine was the first α-agonist tested for treatment of VVS. The Vasovagal Syncope International Study (VASIS),[33] was a large, multicenter, placebo-controlled, double-blinded study that did not show any significant differences in the recurrence of syncope and time for first syncopal episode compared with placebo. Midodrine, a specific α1-agonist, was initially tested in patients with neurogenic orthostatic hypotension.[34] A few clinical trials and a recent meta-analysis assessed the efficacy of midodrine in patients with recurrent

VVS.[34–38] Compared with placebo, midodrine provides beneficial effects in symptom frequency, symptoms during head-up tilt,[34–36] and quality of life.[34,35] A small RCT in pediatric patients also showed a reduction in recurrent syncope.[37]

A recent meta-analysis of 6 randomized clinical trials evaluating α-agonists for treatment of VVS included 329 patients. This meta-analysis reported a large effect favoring midodrine compared with placebo (odds ratio, 0.21; 95% CI, 0.06–0.77; $P = .02$).[38] Weighted mean percentage of responders for midodrine (76.3% ± 7.7%) was significantly higher than that for etilefrine (65.5% ± 15.4%; $P<.001$). The observations reported by this meta-analysis are questionable because of methodological flaws. Nonetheless, there seems to be a significant treatment effect when midodrine is administered and this hypothesis is currently being tested in a large RCT.

Midodrine is reasonably well tolerated, but its use is not recommended in patients with hypertension or heart failure. Midodrine should be administered 3 times per day and titrated to a maximum dose of 40 mg. Despite the lack of strong evidence, midodrine may be indicated in frequently symptomatic VVS patients, refractory to lifestyle measures.

Fludrocortisone

Fludrocortisone is a corticosteroid with marked mineralocorticoid activity that increases sodium and fluid retention and, consequently, intravascular volume expansion. In addition, it upregulates α-adrenergic receptors and may prevent vasodilatation during neurally mediated reflex responses. In spite of the lack of controlled studies, fludrocortisone is often used for the treatment of VVS. A small, randomized, double-blinded, placebo-controlled study showed that 1 g of NaCl in combination with 0.1 mg of fludrocortisone per day plus counseling was ineffective in preventing syncope or presyncope recurrence in children.[39]

The second POST trial (POST II) randomized 213 patients to fludrocortisone or placebo.[40,41] The primary outcome of the study was time to the first recurrence of syncope, which was not significantly reduced by fludrocortisone.[41] The doses of fludrocortisone ranged from 0.1 to 0.4 mg daily. Available evidence does not show a significant reduction in syncope recurrence with fludrocortisone in unselected patients with VVS. Further analysis of the POST II population may identify subgroups that benefit from this therapy.

SSRIs

Increased central serotoninergic activity has been suggested to play a role in sudden inhibition of sympathetic activity, potentially precipitating VVS.[42] Thus, SSRIs have been evaluated in preventing VVS in adults, especially in patients resistant to or intolerant of previous traditional therapies.[42–45]

Fluoxetine was compared with propranolol in a randomized, placebo-controlled study conducted in 94 patients and showed no differences in syncope-free period. A significant improvement in quality of life was observed with fluoxetine.[43]

Paroxetine, another SSRI, was evaluated in a randomized, double-blind, placebo-controlled study in which 68 consecutive patients with recurrent VVS and positive head-up tilt were randomized to paroxetine 20 mg/d or placebo.[44] After 1 month of treatment, the response rates (negative tilt) were 61.8% versus 38.2% ($P<.001$) in the paroxetine and placebo groups, respectively. Paroxetine significantly improved symptoms compared with placebo (17.6% vs 52.9, $P<.0001$).[44]

SSRIs are rarely the first choice in the treatment of neurally mediated reflex syncope. Symptomatic patients in whom standard therapies were ineffective, poorly tolerated, or contraindicated might be prescribed SSRIs, which may be particularly useful in patients with associated anxiety and panic disorders.

Other Inconclusive Treatments

Several other therapeutic strategies for preventions of VVS have been tested, including disopyramide,[45,46] angiotensin-converting enzyme inhibitors,[47,48] erythropoietin,[49] transdermal scopolamine,[50] desmopressin, and implantable drug delivery systems.[1] All of these interventions may be potentially beneficial but the available evidence is limited; these interventions are not recommended for the treatment of recurrent VVS, and should be considered experimental.

SUMMARY

VVS is the most frequent cause of recurrent syncope. Although it has a benign course, quality of life can be severely impaired by recurrent episodes of syncope. Nonpharmacologic measures are simple and usually safe and should be tried as first-line therapy in patients with frequent syncope and no obvious contraindications. Pharmacologic therapy is used and recommended in patients refractory to nonpharmacologic interventions. No specific guidelines are available to indicate which pharmacologic treatment should be initiated; however, in practice, midodrine seems to be the most promising agent and β-blockade may have a role in older patients.

REFERENCES

1. Moya A, Sutton R, Ammirati F, et al. Guidelines for the diagnosis and management of syncope. Eur Heart J 2009;30:2631–71.
2. Mosqueda-Garcia R, Furlan R, Tank J, et al. The elusive pathophysiology of neurally mediated syncope. Circulation 2000;102:2898–906.
3. Wieling W, Colman N, Krediet CT, et al. Non-pharmacological treatment of reflex syncope. Clin Auton Res 2004;14(Suppl 1):62–70.
4. Van Dijk N, Velzeboer S, Destree-Vonk A, et al. Psychological treatment of malignant vasovagal syncope due to blood phobia. Pacing Clin Electrophysiol 2001;24:122–4.
5. Gaggioli G, Bottoni N, Mureddu R, et al. Effects of chronic vasodilator therapy to enhance susceptibility to vasovagal syncope during upright tilt testing. Am J Cardiol 1997;80:1092–4.
6. El-Sayed H, Hainsworth R. Relationship between plasma volume, carotid baroreceptor sensitivity and orthostatic tolerance. Clin Sci (Colch) 1995;88:463–70.
7. El-Sayed H, Hainsworth R. Salt supplement increases plasma volume and orthostatic tolerance in patients with unexplained syncope. Heart 1996;75:134–40.
8. Shichiri M, Tanaka H, Takaya R, et al. Efficacy of high sodium intake in a boy with instantaneous orthostatic hypotension. Clin Auton Res 2002;12:47–50.
9. Wieling W, Van Lieshout JJ, Hainsworth R. Extracellular fluid volume expansion in patients with posturally related syncope. Clin Auton Res 2002;12:242–9.
10. Mtinangi BL, Hainsworth R. Early effects of oral salt on plasma volume, orthostatic tolerance, and baroreceptor sensitivity in patients with syncope. Clin Auton Res 1998;8:231–5.
11. Cariga P, Mathias CJ. Haemodynamics of the pressor effect of oral water in human sympathetic denervation due to autonomic failure. Clin Sci 2001;101:313–9.
12. Jordan J, Shannon JR, Black BK, et al. The pressor response to water drinking in humans. A sympathetic reflex? Circulation 2000;101:504–9.
13. Jordan J, Shannon JR, Grogan E, et al. A potent pressor response elicited by drinking water. Lancet 1999;353:723.
14. Shannon JR, Diedrich A, Biaggioni I, et al. Water drinking as a treatment for orthostatic syndromes. Am J Med 2002;112:355–60.
15. Schroeder C, Bush V, Norcliffe L, et al. Water drinking acutely improves orthostatic tolerance in healthy subjects. Circulation 2002;106:2806–11.
16. Ector H, Reybrouck T, Heidbuchel H, et al. Tilt training: a new treatment for recurrent neurocardiogenic syncope or severe orthostatic intolerance. Pacing Clin Electrophysiol 1998;21:193–6.

17. Abe H, Kondo S, Kohshi K, et al. Usefulness of orthostatic self-training for the prevention of neuro-cardiogenic syncope. Pacing Clin Electrophysiol 2002;25:1454–8.

18. Di Girolamo E, Di Iorio C, Leonzio L, et al. Usefulness of a tilt training program for the prevention of refractory neurocardiogenic syncope in adolescents: a controlled study. Circulation 1999;100:1798–801.

19. Reybrouck T, Heidbüchel H, Van De Werf F, et al. Long-term follow-up results of tilt training therapy in patients with recurrent neurocardiogenic syncope. Pacing Clin Electrophysiol 2002;25:1441–6.

20. Gajek J, Zyśko D, Mazurek W. Efficacy of tilt training in patients with vasovagal syncope. Kardiol Pol 2006;64:602–8.

21. Duygu H, Zoghi M, Turk U, et al. The role of tilt training in preventing recurrent syncope in patients with vasovagal syncope: a prospective and randomized study. Pacing Clin Electrophysiol 2008;31:592–6.

22. Brignole M, Croci F, Menozzi C, et al. Isometric arm counter-pressure maneuvers to abort impending vasovagal syncope. J Am Coll Cardiol 2002;40:2054–60.

23. Krediet P, van Dijk N, Linzer M, et al. Management of vasovagal syncope: controlling or aborting faints by leg crossing and muscle tensing. Circulation 2002;106:1684–9.

24. Van Dijk N, Quartieri F, Blanc JJ, et al. Effectiveness of physical counterpressure maneuvers in preventing vasovagal syncope: the Physical Counterpressure Manoeuvres Trial (PC-Trial). J Am Coll Cardiol 2006;8:1652–7.

25. Romme JJ, Reitsma JB, Go-Schön IK, et al. Prospective evaluation of non-pharmacological treatment in vasovagal syncope. Europace 2010;12:567–73.

26. Brignole M, Menozzi C, Gianfranchi L, et al. A controlled trial of acute and long-term medical therapy in tilt-induced neurally mediated syncope. Am J Cardiol 1992;70:339–42.

27. Sheldon R, Rose S, Flanagan P, et al. Effect of beta blockers on the time to first syncope recurrence in patients after a positive isoproterenol tilt table test. Am J Cardiol 1996;78:536–9.

28. Madrid AH, Ortega J, Rebollo JG, et al. Lack of efficacy of atenolol for the prevention of neurally mediated syncope in a highly symptomatic population: a prospective, double-blind, randomized and placebo-controlled study. J Am Coll Cardiol 2001;37:554–9.

29. Ventura R, Maas R, Zeidler D, et al. A randomized and controlled pilot trial of beta-blockers for the treatment of recurrent syncope in patients with a positive or negative response to head-up tilt test. Pacing Clin Electrophysiol 2002;25:816–21.

30. Flevari P, Livanis EG, Theodorakis GN, et al. Vasovagal syncope: a prospective, randomized, crossover evaluation of the effect of propranolol, nadolol and placebo on syncope recurrence and patients' well-being. J Am Coll Cardiol 2002;40:499–504.

31. Sheldon R, Connolly S, Rose S, et al. Prevention of Syncope Trial (POST): a randomized, placebo-controlled study of metoprolol in the prevention of vasovagal syncope. Circulation 2006;113:1164–70.

32. Sheldon RS, Morillo CA, Klingenheben T, et al. Age-dependent effect of beta blockers in preventing vasovagal syncope. Circ Arrhythm Electrophysiol 2012;5(5):920–6.

33. Raviele A, Brignole M, Sutton R, et al. Effect of etilefrine in preventing syncopal recurrence in patients with vasovagal syncope: a double-blind, randomized, placebo-controlled trial. The Vasovagal Syncope International Study. Circulation 1999;99:1452–7.

34. Ward CR, Gray JC, Gilroy JJ, et al. Midodrine: a role in the management of neurocardiogenic syncope. Heart 1998;79:45–9.

35. Perez-Lugones A, Schweikert R, Pavia S, et al. Usefulness of midodrine in patients with severely symptomatic neurocardiogenic syncope: a randomized control study. J Cardiovasc Electrophysiol 2001;12:935–8.

36. Kaufmann H, Saadia D, Voustianiouk A. Midodrine in neurally mediated syncope: a double-blind, randomized, crossover study. Ann Neurol 2002;52:342–5.

37. Zhang QY, Du JB, Tang CS. The efficacy of midodrine hydrochloride in the treatment of children with vasovagal syncope. J Pediatr 2006;149:777–80.

38. Liao Y, Li X, Zhang Y, et al. α-Adrenoceptor agonists for the treatment of vasovagal syncope: a meta-analysis of worldwide published data. Acta Paediatr 2009;98:1194–2000.

39. Salim MA, Di Sessa TG. Effectiveness of fludrocortisone and salt in preventing syncope recurrence in children: a double blind, placebo-controlled, randomized trial. J Am Coll Cardiol 2005;45:484–8.

40. Raj SR, Rose S, Ritchie D, et al. The Second Prevention of Syncope Trial (POST II): a randomized clinical trial of fludrocortisone for the prevention of neurally mediated syncope: rationale and study design. Am Heart J 2006;151:1186.e11–7.

41. Sheldon R, Morillo CA, Krahn A, et al. A randomized clinical trial of fludrocortisone for the prevention of vasovagal syncope (POST2). Can J Cardiol 2011;27:S335–6.

42. Grubb BP, Samoil D, Kosinski D, et al. Use of sertraline hydrochloride in the treatment of refractory neurocardiogenic syncope in children and adolescents. J Am Coll Cardiol 1994;24:490–4.

43. Theodorakis GN, Leftheriotis D, Livanis EG, et al. Fluoxetine vs. propranolol in the treatment of vasovagal syncope: a prospective, randomized, placebo-controlled study. Europace 2006;8:193–8.

44. Di Girolamo E, Di Iorio C, Sabatini P, et al. Effects of paroxetine hydrochloride, a selective serotonin reuptake inhibitor, on refractory vasovagal

syncope: a randomized, double-blind, placebo-controlled study. J Am Coll Cardiol 1999;33:1227–30.

45. Milstein S, Buetikofer J, Dunnigan A, et al. Usefulness of disopyramide for prevention of upright tilt-induced hypotension-bradycardia. Am J Cardiol 1990;65:1339–944.

46. Morillo CA, Leitch JW, Yee R, et al. A placebo-controlled trial of intravenous and oral disopyramide for prevention of neurally mediated syncope induced by head-up tilt. J Am Coll Cardiol 1993;22:1843–8.

47. Zeng CY, Zhu Z, Liu G, et al. Inhibitory effect of enalapril on neurally mediated syncope in elderly patients. J Cardiovasc Pharmacol 1998; 31:638–42.

48. Zeng C, Zhu Z, Liu G, et al. Randomized, double-blind, placebo-controlled trial of oral enalapril in patients with neurally mediated syncope. Am Heart J 1998;136:852–8.

49. Kawakami K, Abe H, Harayama N, et al. Successful treatment of severe orthostatic hypotension with erythropoietin. Pacing Clin Electrophysiol 2003;2:105–7.

50. Lee TM, Su SF, Chen MF, et al. Usefulness of transdermal scopolamine for vasovagal syncope. Am J Cardiol 1996;78:480–2.

Pacemaker Therapy in Syncope

Angel Moya, MD, PhD*, Ivo Roca-Luque, MD,
Jaume Francisco-Pascual, MD, Jordi Perez-Rodón, MD,
Nuria Rivas, MD

KEYWORDS

- Pacemaker therapy • Syncope • Asystole • Bradycardia • Tachycardia • Bundle branch block
- Neurally mediated or reflex

KEY POINTS

- In patients with neurally mediated syncope, current syncope guidelines recommend pacing only for adult patients (>40 years old according to inclusion criteria of different pacing trials for neurally mediated syncope) with recurrent syncope and documented cardioinhibition during spontaneous syncope.
- Some questions remain without clear answers in this field; for example, the better pacing mode (with an increasing role of closed loop pacemakers) and the role of adenosine-5' triphosphate testing in predicting patients with asystole during syncope.
- The management of patients with syncope and bundle branch block has some unanswered questions.
- Based on the risk of paroxysmal atrioventricular block but also because another possible mechanisms of syncope exist (ie, ventricular arrhythmias), 2 strategies are possible, both of which are accepted in the guidelines. One strategy is direct implantation of a pacemaker. The other is a more conservative strategy based on a stepwise approach with EPS and ILR if negative.

INTRODUCTION

According to current guidelines,[1] syncope is defined as a transient loss of consciousness caused by transient cerebral hypoperfusion. Transient cerebral hypoperfusion can be due to a decrease in peripheral resistance, usually because of vasodilatation, or a decrease in cardiac output, that can be secondary to an obstructive cardiac disease or to an arrhythmia, either bradycardia or tachycardia.

Pacemaker implantation is clearly indicated when bradycardia can be documented during syncope and is secondary to sinus node dysfunction or to atrioventricular (AV) block (**Tables 1** and **2**).[2,3]

Nevertheless, in many occasions, although a bradycardia can be suspected on either clinical or electrocardiographic (ECG) findings, there is no clear correlation between syncope and arrhythmia. In addition, there are many situations (ie, reflex syncope) in which the mechanism is mixed with bradycardia and vasodilatation, and it is not clear

in these patients if treating the bradycardia with cardiac stimulation prevents syncope recurrence.

In this article, those aspects not clearly solved about pacing therapy in syncope are discussed.

Neurally Mediated Syncope

Introduction

The term reflex syncope or neurally mediated syncope is usually applied to an heterogeneous group of conditions in which cardiovascular reflexes that are normally useful in controlling the circulation become intermittently inappropriate, in response to a trigger, resulting in vasodilatation and/or bradycardia and thereby in a drop in blood pressure, finally leading to a transient global cerebral hypoperfusion (**Fig. 1**).[1] According to this definition and considering the pattern of response to tilt testing, reflex syncope was classified as vasodepressor, mixed, or cardioinhibitory.[4]

Unitat Arrítmies, Hospital Universitari Vall d'Hebrón, Universitat Autònoma de Barcelona, Barcelona, Spain
* Corresponding author. Hospital Vall d'Hebron, P. Vall d'Hebron 119-129, Barcelona 08035, Spain.
E-mail address: amoya@vhebron.net

Cardiol Clin 31 (2013) 131–142
http://dx.doi.org/10.1016/j.ccl.2012.10.001
0733-8651/13/$ – see front matter © 2013 Elsevier Inc. All rights reserved.

Table 1
Pacing recommendations for patients with syncope and bundle branch block

ESC Pacing Guidelines 2007	ACC/AHA/HRS Pacing Guidelines 2008	ESC Syncope Guidelines 2009
Class I		
• Intermittent third-degree atrioventricular block *(Level of Evidence: C)* • Second-degree Mobitz II atrioventricular block *(Level of Evidence: C)* • Alternating bundle branch block *(Level of evidence C)* • Findings on electrophysiologic study of markedly prolonged HV interval (HV ≥ 100 ms) or pacing-induced infra-His block in patients with symptoms *(Level of Evidence: C)*	• Permanent pacemaker implantation is indicated for advanced second-degree AV block or intermittent third-degree AV block *(Level of Evidence: B)* • Permanent pacemaker implantation is indicated for type II second-degree AV block *(Level of Evidence: B)* • Permanent pacemaker implantation is indicated for alternating bundle-branch block *(Level of Evidence: C)*	• Pacing is indicated in patients with syncope and second-degree Mobitz II, advanced or complete AV block *(Level of Evidence: B)* • Pacing is indicated in patients with syncope, BBB, and positive EPS[a] *(Level of Evidence: B)*
Class IIa		
• Syncope not demonstrated to be due to atrioventricular block when other likely causes have been excluded, specifically ventricular tachycardia *(Level of Evidence: B)* • Neuromuscular diseases (eg, myotonic muscular dystrophy, Kearns-Sayre syndrome, etc) with any degree of fascicular block *(Level of Evidence: C)* • Incidental findings on electrophysiologic study of markedly prolonged HV interval (HV ≥ 100 ms) or pacing-induced infra-His block in patients without symptoms *(Level of Evidence: C)*	• Permanent pacemaker implantation is reasonable for syncope not demonstrated to be due to AV block when other likely causes have been excluded, specifically ventricular tachycardia (VT). *(Level of Evidence: B)* • Permanent pacemaker implantation is reasonable for an incidental finding at electrophysiologic study of a markedly prolonged HV interval (greater than or equal to 100 ms) in asymptomatic patients *(Level of Evidence: B)* • Permanent pacemaker implantation is reasonable for an incidental finding at electrophysiologic study of pacing-induced infra-His block that is not physiologic *(Level of Evidence: B)*	• Pacing should be considered in patients with unexplained syncope and BBB *(Level of Evidence: C)*
Class IIb		
None	• Permanent pacemaker implantation may be considered in the setting of neuromuscular diseases such as myotonic muscular dystrophy, Erb dystrophy (limb-girdle muscular dystrophy), and peroneal muscular atrophy with bifascicular block or any fascicular block, with or without symptoms *(Level of Evidence: C)*	None

(continued on next page)

Table 1
(continued)

ESC Pacing Guidelines 2007	ACC/AHA/HRS Pacing Guidelines 2008	ESC Syncope Guidelines 2009
Class III		
• Bundle branch block without atrioventricular block or symptoms *(Level of Evidence: B)* • Bundle branch block with first-degree atrioventricular block without symptoms *(Level of Evidence: B)*	• Permanent pacing is not indicated for fascicular block without AV block or symptoms *(Level of Evidence: B)* • Permanent pacing is not indicated for fascicular block with first-degree AV block without symptoms *(Level of Evidence: B)*	Pacing is not indicated in patients with unexplained syncope with any evidence of any conduction disturbance *(Level of Evidence: C)*

^a Positive EPS in patients with syncope and BBB in the ESC Syncope guidelines: Baseline interval HV $\geq$100 ms or second- or third-degree His-Purkinge block during incremental atrial pacing or with pharmacologic challenge (*Class of recommendation I, Level of Evidence B*), HV interval between 70 and 100 ms (*Class of recommendation IIa, Level of Evidence B*).

Table 2
Pacing recommendations for neuro-mediated syncope

ESC Pacing Guidelines 2007	ACC/AHA/HRS Pacing Guidelines 2008	ESC Syncope Guidelines 2009
Class I		
None	None	None
Class IIa		
Patients over 40 y of age with recurrent severe vasovagal syncope who show prolonged asystole during ECG recording and/or tilt testing, after failure of other therapeutic options and being informed of the conflicting results of trials *(Level of Evidence: C)*	None	Cardiac pacing should be considered in patients with frequent recurrent reflex syncope, age >40 y, and documented spontaneous cardioinhibitory response during monitoring *(Level of Evidence: B)*
Class IIb		
Patients under 40 y of age with recurrent severe vasovagal syncope who show prolonged asystole during ECG recording and/or tilt testing, after failure of other therapeutic options and being informed of the conflicting results of trials *(Level of Evidence: C)*	Permanent pacing may be considered for significantly symptomatic neurocardiogenic syncope associated with bradycardia documented spontaneously or at the time of tilt-table testing *(Level of Evidence: B)*	Cardiac pacing should be indicated in patients with tilt-induced cardioinhibitory response with frequent unpredictable syncope and age >40 y after alternative therapy has failed *(Level of Evidence: C)*
Class III		
Patients without demonstrable bradycardia during reflex syncope *(Level of Evidence: C)*	Permanent pacing is not indicated for situational vasovagal syncope in which avoidance behavior is effective and preferred *(Level of Evidence: C)*	Cardiac pacing is not indicated in the absence of a documented cardioinhibitory reflex *(Level of Evidence: A)*

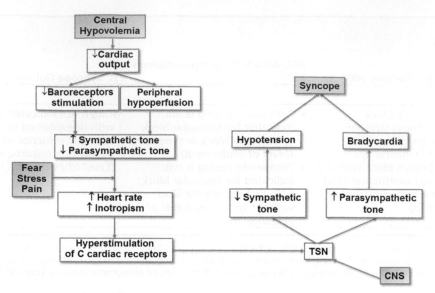

Fig. 1. Syncope pathophysiology. CNS, Central nervous system; STN, solitary tract nucleus.

In the presence of predominantly vasodepressor response, there is no role for pacemaker therapy (**Fig. 2**). The question arises in those patients who have a cardioinhibitory component, especially those with a prolonged asystole.

However, several questions must be stressed in this field. First, neurally mediated syncope is a benign disease that usually presents in young people and that has an erratic course, appearing usually in clusters with long periods of remission.

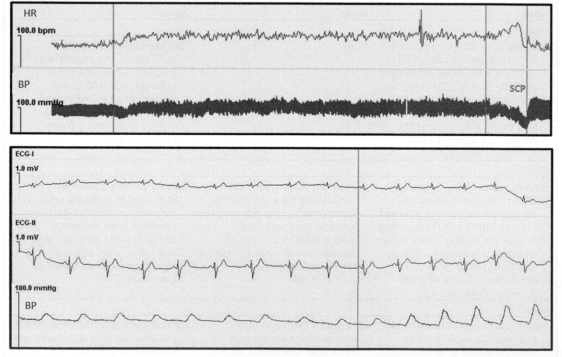

Fig. 2. Tilt test recording register of vasodepressor syncope. A drop in arterial blood pressure without an initial increase in heart rate can be seen during tilt test, followed, at the time of minimal arterial blood pressure, by a minimal drop in heart rate; significant heart rate decrease during the syncope. (*Top*, summary of the tilt test recording; *bottom*, detail of arterial blood pressure and ECG).

Accordingly, cautious must be taken in implanting a pacemaker in the young population for such condition. The second main problem is the fact that, as previously stated when defining reflex or neurally mediated syncope, the cardioinhibitory response, even in the presence of severe asystole (usually >3 seconds), is only one of the components of the mechanism, as a vasodepressor reaction is always present and usually appears earlier in the development of syncope (**Fig. 3**).[5] Consequently, treating bradycardia with a pacemaker can be insufficient in preventing syncope in some of these patients.

Historical Aspects

The role of treating bradycardia in neurally mediated syncope has attracted the interest of researchers for many years. Sir Thomas Lewis in 1931[6] administered atropine in patients during a "vasovagal" syncope and described that: "While raising the pulse rate up to and beyond normal levels during the attack, leaves the blood pressure below normal and the patient still pale and not fully conscious." With the use of tilt testing, several authors analyzed the role of pacing in preventing syncope induced during tilt testing. Although it was clear that single-chamber ventricular pacing did not prevent syncope recurrence,[7,8] it was suggested that dual-chamber pacing could be useful in delaying or avoiding reflex syncope induced during tilt testing.[9,10] However, it has been shown that responses observed during tilt testing did not predict clinical outcome.

Controlled Studies

Nonblinded studies based on tilt testing findings

In the late 1990s, several studies were published analyzing the role of the pacemaker in patients with suspected neurally mediated syncope, that is, patients without structural heart disease and with normal ECG.[11–13] The inclusion criteria varied from different studies (**Table 3**), but the patients were selected according to the response observed during tilt testing. Included patients were randomized to pacemaker implantation or no specific therapy in 2 studies[11,12] or to beta-blockers in another study[13] that at that time was considered the best medical treatment. In all 3 studies (total, 189 patients), patients in whom a pacemaker was implanted had less syncopal recurrences (10%–25% recurrences in pacemaker group and 75%–90% in nonpacemaker group) than those without a pacemaker (**Fig. 4**).

Blinded studies based on tilt testing findings

One of the criticisms of those studies[11–13] was the fact that they were not blinded. In this sense, a possible expected effect of implanting a pacemaker, rather than pacing itself, could play a role in preventing syncope recurrences.[14]

To avoid this possible bias, and considering that after these initial studies there were data suggesting that a pacemaker could be useful, new blinded studies were performed.[15–17] In these trials, all patients who fulfilled inclusion criteria received a pacemaker and were randomized to pacemaker

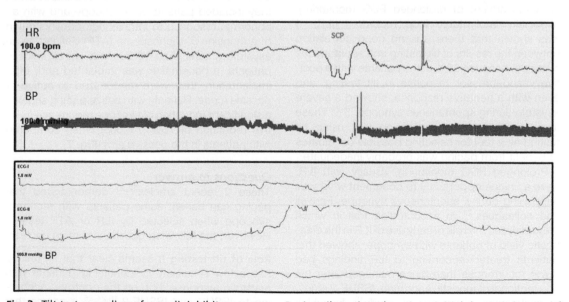

Fig. 3. Tilt test recording of a cardioinhibitory syncope. During tilt testing, there is an initial decrease in arterial blood pressure that is followed by a progressive bradycardia and a severe asystole during syncope. (*Top*, summary of the tilt test recording; *bottom*, detail of arterial blood pressure and ECG.)

Table 3
Inclusion criteria and mode of pacing in studies based on tilt testing findings

| Trial | Inclusion Criteria | | Mode of Pacing in Active Arm |
	Number of Syncopes	TT Response	
VPS[11]	6 in all live	HR <60,70,80 bpm	DDI
VASIS[12]	3 in 2 y	HR <40 bpm or asystole >3 s	DDR-RDR
SYDIT[13]	3 in 2 y	HR <60 bpm	DDR-RDR
VPS II[15]	6 in all live	HR × AP < 6000	DDR-RDR
SYNPACE[16]	6 in all live	HR <60 bpm or asystole >3 s	DDR-RDR
INVASY[17]	2 in a y	Cardioinhibitory or mixt	DDDR-CLS

Abbreviations: AP, arterial pressure; HR, heart rate; TT, tilt test.

ON or OFF. In 2 of these studies,[15,16] syncope recurrence was the same irrespective of the activation of pacemaker, suggesting that pacing was not useful in preventing cardioinhibitory syncope. Only in one of these studies, in which a pacemaker with closed loop stimulation algorithm was used (INOS[2], Biotronik), patients allocated to the pacemaker ON arm showed a reduction of syncope recurrence when compared with those in the pacemaker OFF arm.[17] In this algorithm, pacing is triggered by variations in myocardial contractility despite changes in heart rate. In this study, despite being a randomized trial, there were only 9 patients in the pacemaker ON arm and 50 in the pacemaker OFF arm, limiting the validity of analysis (**Fig. 5**).

Controlled studies based other selection criteria

With the advent of prolonged ECG monitoring, especially implantable loop recorders (ILR), it was shown that there was no good correlation between the results of tilt testing and spontaneous syncope, because 50% of the patients with a positive vasodepressor response in tilt testing, and even with a negative response, showed a severe asystole during spontaneous syncope.[18–20] These findings lead to the perception that using tilt testing as a tool for selecting possible candidates to benefit from pacing was probably inadequate.

Prolonged ECG monitoring, usually with ILR, gave a unique opportunity to document what was happening during spontaneous syncope. Farwell and colleagues,[21] in a controlled trial in which they analyzed the role of early use of ILR in the diagnostic yield of patients with syncope, showed that patients treated according to ILR findings had fewer recurrences than those managed after the conventional diagnostic approach. ISSUE-2 study, a multicenter observational study[19] in which patients were treated according to ILR findings, also confirmed that a strategy based on early

diagnostic ILR application, with therapy delayed until documentation of syncope, allows a safe, specific, and effective therapy in patients with neurally mediated syncope. According to this, a controlled multicenter prospective double-blind study[22] in which patients with neurally mediated syncope and documented spontaneous asystole (>3 seconds with symptoms or >6 seconds without symptoms) with ILR recording, received a dual-chamber pacemaker with rate drop response algorithm, was implanted and were randomized to pacing or sensing mode (pacing OFF). Patients on the active dual-chamber pacing arm showed a reduction of syncope recurrences when compared with patients with a pacemaker programmed in sensing mode (relative risk reduction, 57%; absolute risk reduction, 32%; P<.005) (**Fig. 6**). Recently, Flammang and colleagues[23] published a double-blind randomized trial in which they included patients with syncope and with an abnormal response to intravenous administration of adenosine-5′ triphosphate (ATP) defined as an asystole greater than 10 seconds. In all elective patients, a pacemaker was implanted and, after implantation, they were randomized to active or passive mode. Patients with active pacing showed a significant reduction of syncope recurrence (relative reduction of 75%; P<.005) when compared with patients in the passive arm (**Fig. 7**).

Questions to answer

These 2 recent articles[22,23] demonstrated that pacing can benefit some patients with recurrent syncope when selected by ILR or ATP testing. However, the following questions remain unclear.

Role of tilt testing It seems clear that tilt testing has a low sensitivity in identifying patients with asystolic response, but, on the contrary, according to ISSUE and ISSUE-2,[18,24,25] it seems that an asystolic response observed during tilt testing is very specific (75%–80% positive predictive

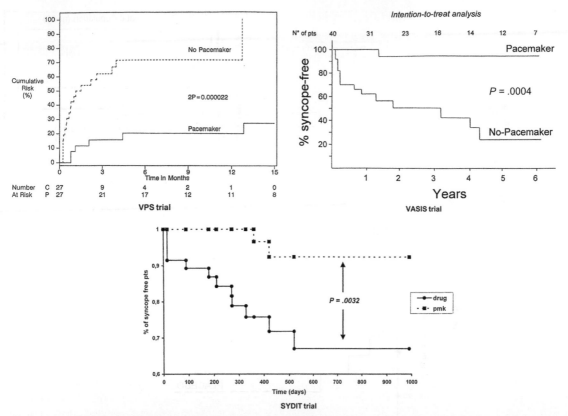

Fig. 4. Controlled nonblinded studies based on tilt testing findings. *Left*: VPS trial Kaplan-Meier plots of the time to the first recurrence of syncope among 27 patients randomized to receive a pacemaker and 27 patients randomized not to receive a pacemaker by intention-to-treat analysis. *Right*: VASIS trial. Kaplan-Meier estimates of the probability of remaining free of syncopal recurrences in 19 patients in the pacemaker arm and 23 patients in the no-pacemaker arm in the intention-to-treat analysis. *Down*: SYDIT trial. Kaplan-Meier estimation of the probability of remaining free of syncopal recurrences in 46 patients in the pacemaker arm and 47 patients in the pharmacologic arm in the intention-to-treat analysis. (*From* [*Left*] Connolly SJ, Sheldon R, Roberts RS, et al. The North American Vasovagal Pacemaker Study (VPS). A randomized trial of permanent cardiac pacing for the prevention of vasovagal syncope. J Am Coll Cardiol 1999;33:16–20; with permission; [*Right*] Sutton R, Brignole M, Menozzi C, et al. Dual-chamber pacing in the treatment of neutrally mediated tilt-positive cardioinhibitory syncope: pacemaker versus no therapy: a multicenter randomized study. The Vasovagal Syncope Internation Study (VASIS). Circulation 2000;102:294–9; with permission; and [*Down*] Ammirati F, Colivicchi F, Santini M, et al. Permanent cardiac pacing vs medical treatment for the prevention of recurrent vasovagal syncope: a multicenter, randomized, controlled trial. Circulation 2001;104:52–7; with permission.)

value) of an asystole during spontaneous syncope. Further analysis of the correlation between tilt testing and spontaneous syncope in ISSUE-3 will help in answering this question.

Age Most of the studies did not include a young population in an attempt to avoid pacing in young patients. In ISSUE-2 and ISSUE-3 studies,[19,22] patients had to be 40 years old minimum old to be included (mean age, ISSUE-2, >65 years, ISSUE-3, 63 years and older) and, although in the study of Flammang and colleagues[23] patients greater than or equal to 18 years old could be included, mean age was also higher (>75 years). These data support that pacemaker should be indicated mainly in patients with advanced age,

but there are no data in younger patients with very recurrent syncope.

ATP testing In the study of Flammang and colleagues,[23] patients were selected according to the response to ATP testing. Previous studies[15,24,25] in patients with syncope of unknown origin and positive response to ATP testing showed a poor correlation between the response to ATP and spontaneous syncope documented by ILR. Most recently,[26] it has been suggested that those patients who have a positive response to ATP represent a specific group of patients with a specific purinergic profile that manifests clinically with syncope without minimal prodromal symptoms[27] and sudden AV block

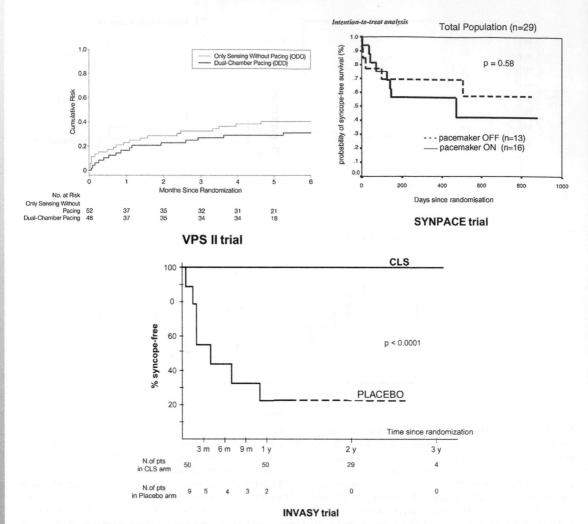

VPS II trial

SYNPACE trial

INVASY trial

Fig. 5. Controlled blinded studies based on tilt testing findings. *Left*: VPS II trial. Kaplan-Meier plots of the time to the first recurrence of syncope among 52 patients randomized to the pacemaker programmed to only sensing mode and 43 patients randomized to dual chamber pacing mode. *Middle*: SYNPACE trial. Kaplan–Meier estimates of the probability of remaining free of syncopal recurrences in 13 patients with pacemaker OFF and in 16 patients with pacemaker ON. *Right*: INVASY trial. Probability of remaining free of syncopal recurrences (Kaplan-Meier estimation) in 41 patients in the CLS arm and in 9 patients in the control group. (*From [Left]* Sheldon R, Connolly S; Vasovagal Pacemaker Study II. Second Vasovagal Pacemaker Study (VPS II): rationale, design, results, and implications for practice and future clinical trials. Card Electrophysiol Rev. 2003 Dec;7(4):411–5; with permission; *[Middle]* Raviele A, Gliada F, Menozzi C, et al. A randomized, double-blind, placebo-controlled study of permanent cardiac pacing for the treatment of recurrent tilt-induced vasovagal syncope. The vasovagal syncope and pacing trial (SYNPACE). Eur Heart J 2004;25:1741–8; with permission; and *[Right]* Occhetta E, Bortnik M, Audogilio R, et al. Closed loop stimulation in prevention of vasovagal syncope. Inotropy controlled pacing in vasovagal syncope (INVASY): a multicentre randomized, single blind, controlled study. Europace 2004;6:538–47; with permission.)

rather than the progressive sinus bradycardia observed typically in reflex syncope.[28] In summary, although recent publications suggest a role of ATP testing in predicting asystole in these patients, the issue remains controversial.

Mode of pacing Different pacing modes have been programmed in the different trials. In the

study of Flammang,[23] in patients in the active group, pacemakers were programmed at DDD mode (dual-chamber pacing) at 70 bpm, whereas in ISSUE-3,[22] a pacemaker with a rate drop response algorithm was implanted. Both studies were not designed to analyze which pacing mode was better in preventing syncope recurrences. In addition, some authors have suggested that

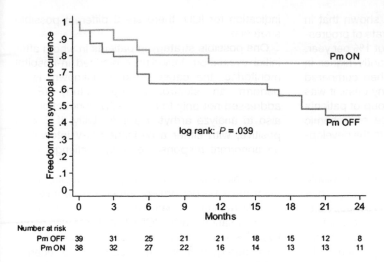

Fig. 6. ISSUE 3 TRIAL: Kaplan–Meier estimates of the probability of remaining free of syncopal recurrences in 39 patients with pacemaker OFF and in 38 patients with pacemaker on. (*From* Brignole M, Menozzi C, Moya A, et al. Pacemaker therapy in patients with neutrally mediated syncope and documented asystole: Third International Study on Syncope of Uncertain Etiology (ISSUE-3): a randomized trial. Circulation 2012;29:2566–71; with permission.)

pacing based on closed-loop stimulation[17,29] can be better to prevent syncope than other pacing modes. During neurally mediated syncope, an increase in myocardial contractility associated with a reduction of ventricular filling produces an increase in baroreceptor afferent flow and a consequent decrease in the heart rate. Closed-loop stimulation pacemakers monitor variations in right ventricular intracardiac impedance. In this sense this pacing mode begins to pace earlier than other pacing modes, at the initial phases of the neurally mediated reaction before bradycardia. Until large well-designed studies are published confirming this hypothesis, these data must be considered preliminary.

SYNCOPE AND BUNDLE BRANCH BLOCK

The presence of bundle branch block (BBB) is a marker of increased risk for paroxysmal or progression to complete AV block, but it is not itself a diagnostic finding.

By analyzing several series of patients with syncope and BBB, it has been observed that on average 50% of these patients have some type of structural heart disease.[30–33]

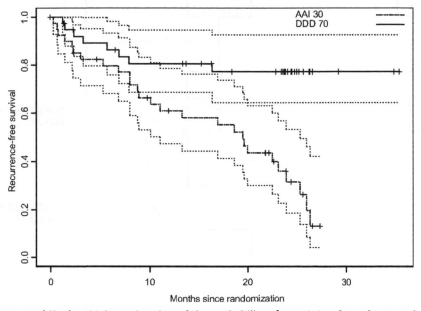

Fig. 7. Flammang et al Kaplan–Meier estimation of the probability of remaining free of syncopal recurrences in 30 patients with pacemaker in AAI mode and in 70 patients with pacemaker in DDD mode. (*From* Flammang D, Church TR, De Roy L, et al. Treatment of unexplained syncope: a multicenter, randomized trial of cardiac pacing guided by adenosine 5'-triphosphate testing. Circulation 2012;125:31–6; with permission.)

More than 20 years ago it was shown that in patients with bifascicular BBB, the rate of progression to complete AV block was about 1% per year, and this progression was significantly higher in patients with previous syncope when compared with asymptomatic patients.[34] In any case, it was also shown that mortality in this group of patients was more related to the presence of ischemic heart disease and heart failure than to the development of AV block.

By considering all the data, patients with syncope and BBB are not only at risk of AV block, but they can also have reflex syncope or syncope due to a tachyarrhythmia, or even the syncope can be the first manifestation of some previously asymptomatic structural heart disease. In this sense, in every patient with syncope and BBB, a comprehensive cardiac evaluation including echocardiography should be performed. If, according to clinical evaluation, and specifically echocardiography evaluation, the patient fulfills criteria for implantable cardiac defibrillator (ICD), it should be implanted. In those cases in which the patient does not have underlying structural heart disease or at least they do not have an

indication for ICD, there are 2 different possible strategies.

One possible strategy in patients in whom after initial evaluation, including prolonged in-hospital monitoring, the cause remains unknown, is to perform an electrophysiologic study (EPS), addressed not only to analyze AV conduction but also to analyze arrhythmia inducibility. If EPS is positive, with either a prolonged H-V interval or an abnormal response to drug challenge, data suggestive of sinus node dysfunction, or if an arrhythmia is induced, appropriate specific treatment must be performed: either a pacemaker or tachyarrhythmia treatment, respectively (with drugs, ablation, and/or ICD). In patients with negative EPS, implantation of an ILR can be indicated. This strategy has proven to be safe in a recently published prospective observational study[33] and helps to identify those patients who have syncope caused by other etiologies than bradycardia, such as ventricular arrhythmias or nonarrhythmic syncope (**Fig. 8**).

On the other hand, another commonly accepted, more straightforward strategy could be to implant a pacemaker directly, because of

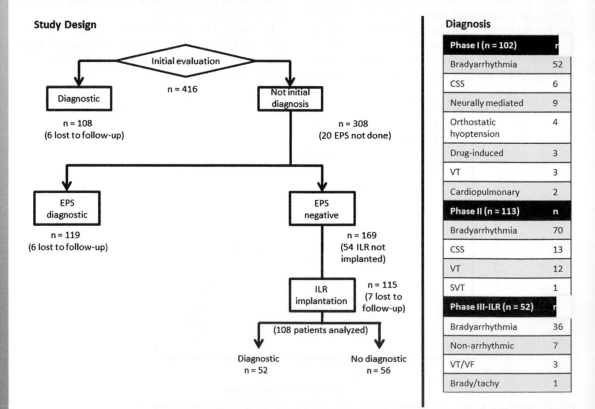

Fig. 8. Study design and diagnoses found in B4 trial. CCS, Carotid sinus syncope; SVT, supraventricular tachycardia; VT, ventricular tachycardia. (*From* Moya A, García-Civera R, Croci F, et al. Diagnosis, management, and outcomes of patients with syncope and bundle branch block. Eur Heart J 2011;32:1535–41; with permission.)

the risk of paroxysmal AV block as the cause of syncope in this group of patients.

In fact, both strategies are considered currently to be class IIa recommendations in the guidelines.[1,2]

Whether one strategy is better or most cost-effective than the other remains unanswered today. A prospective controlled trial that will compare both strategies is ongoing.[35]

SUMMARY

Pacing therapy is an accepted therapy for patients with syncope with documented bradyarrhythmia. However, there are 2 groups of patients with some controversial issues that have been discussed in this article.

Patients with neurally mediated syncope were discussed first. In this group of patients, the role of pacing is only recommended by the current syncope guidelines for adult patients (>40 years old according to inclusion criteria of different pacing trials for neurally mediated syncope) with recurrent syncope and documented cardioinhibition during spontaneous syncope. Some questions remain without a clear answer in this field, like the better pacing mode (with and increasing role of closed loop pacemakers) and the role of ATP testing in predicting patients with asystole during syncope.

Finally, the management of patients with syncope and BBB remains with some unanswered questions. In these patients, both the risk of paroxysmal AV block and also the existence of other possible mechanisms of syncope (ie, ventricular arrhythmias) are possible. In this sense, the decision of direct implantation of a pacemaker and also a strategy more conservatively based on a stepwise approach with EPS and ILR if negative are accepted in the guidelines.

The ongoing randomized trials will help us improve the management of these patients.

REFERENCES

1. Moya A, Sutton R, Ammirati F, et al. Guidelines for the diagnosis and management of syncope. Eur Heart J 2009;30:2631–71.
2. Vardas PE, Auricchio A, Blanc JJ, et al. Guidelines for cardiac pacing and cardiac resynchronization therapy. Eur Heart J 2007;28:2256–95.
3. Epstein AE, DiMarco JP, Ellenbogen KA, et al. ACC/AHA/HRS 2008 guidelines for device-based therapy of cardiac rhythm abnormalities. J Am Coll Cardiol 2008;53:e1–62.
4. Sutton R, Petersen M, Brignole M, et al. Proposed classification for tilt induced vasovagal syncope. Eur J Cardiac Pacing Electrophysiol 1992;3:180–3.
5. Alboni P, Alboni M, Bertorelle G. The origin of vasovagal syncope: to protect the heart or to escape predation? Clin Auton Res 2008;18:170–8.
6. Lewis T. A lecture on vasovagal syncope and carotid sinus mechanism. BMJ 1932;1:873–6.
7. Fitzpatrick AP, Travill CM, Vadas PE, et al. Recurrent symptoms after ventricular pacing in unexplained syncope. Pacing Clin Electrophysiol 1990;13:619–24.
8. Samoil D, Grubb BP. Vasovagal syncope: current concepts in diagnosis and treatment. Heart Dis Stroke 1993;2:247–9.
9. Fitzpatrick A, Theodorakis G, Ahmed R, et al. Dual chamber pacing aborts vasovagal syncope induced by head-up 60 degrees tilt. Pacing Clin Electrophysiol 1991;14:13–9.
10. Petersen ME, Chamberlain-Webber R, Fitzpatrick AP, et al. Permanent pacing for cardioinhibitory malignant vasovagal syndrome. Br Heart J 1994;71:274–81.
11. Connolly SJ, Sheldon R, Roberts RS, et al. The North American Vasovagal Pacemaker Study (VPS). A randomized trial of permanent cardiac pacing for the prevention of vasovagal syncope. J Am Coll Cardiol 1999;33:16–20.
12. Sutton R, Brignole M, Menozzi C, et al. Dual-chamber pacing in the treatment of neutrally mediated tilt-positive cardioinhibitory syncope: pacemaker versus no therapy: a multicenter randomized study the Vasovagal Syncope Internation Study (VASIS). Circulation 2000;102:294–9.
13. Ammirati F, Colivicchi F, Santini M, et al. Permanent cardiac pacing versus medical treatment for the prevention of recurrent vasovagal syncope: a multicenter, randomized, controlled trial. Circulation 2001;104:52–7.
14. Sud S, Massel D, Klein GJ, et al. The expectation effect and cardiac pacing for refractory vasovagal syncope. Am J Med 2007;120:54–62.
15. Connolly SJ, Sheldon R, Thorpe KE, et al. Pacemaker therapy for prevention of syncope in patients with recurrent severe vasovagal syncope: second asovagal Pacemaker Studi (VPS II): a randomized trial. JAMA 2003;289:2224–9.
16. Raviele A, Gliada F, Menozzi C, et al. A randomized, double-blind, placebo-controlled study of permanent cardiac pacing for the treatment of recurrent tilt-induced vasovagal syncope. The vasovagal syncope and pacing trial (SYNPACE). Eur Heart J 2004;25:1741–8.
17. Occhetta E, Bortnik M, Audogilio R, et al. Closed loop stimulation in prevention of vasovagal syncope. Inotropy Controlled Pacing in Vasovagal Syncope (INVASY): a multicentre randomized, single blind, controlled study. Europace 2004;6:538–47.
18. Moya A, Brignole M, Menozzi C, et al. Mechanism of syncope in patients with isolated syncope and in patients with tilt-positive syncope. Circulation 2001; 104:1261–7.

> **Box 1**
> **Syncope 2020: 5 grand challenges**
>
> - Learn the cause and integrated physiology of vasovagal syncope by 2020.
> - Develop at least 1 effective treatment of moderately frequent vasovagal syncope in patients without complications by 2020.
> - Develop at least 1 effective treatment of vasovagal syncope in patients with confounding comorbidities such as hypertension by 2020.
> - Reduce yearly health care spending on syncope by 25% while improving the diagnosis rate and patient satisfaction by 2020.
> - Develop an individualized approach to most patients with syncope by 2020.

and is worsened by difficulties with patient enrollment and with contractual and regulatory requirements in most countries. Nonetheless, these are critical gaps that must be assessed.

Grand challenge 2: Develop at least 1 effective treatment of moderately frequent vasovagal syncope in patients without complications by 2020.

Grand challenge 3: Develop at least 1 effective treatment of vasovagal syncope in patients with confounding comorbidities such as hypertension by 2020.

HEALTH SERVICES DELIVERY

The articles by Win Shen, Giorgio Costantino, and their colleagues testify that our current health services approach to syncope is incoherent, ineffective, expensive, and usually flies in the face of what is known to work and is appropriate. Too many patients undergo electroencephalography, brain imaging, assessment for coronary artery disease, and imaging for syncope in low-risk settings. Most of these investigations are known to have a low rate of diagnostic yield. Tilt tests are used often when a good history would suffice. Simply applying what is now known could prevent most of this, but despite many intelligent attempts, ways to streamline care and make it more accurate have not been found. Innovative knowledge translation strategies using both old and new techniques might improve our delivery of care; this has the potential to save several billion dollars (and euros) yearly.

Grand challenge 4: Reduce yearly health care spending on syncope by 25% while improving diagnosis rate and patient satisfaction by 2020.

INDIVIDUALIZED APPROACH TO SYNCOPE

There are multiple paths to syncope, and our assessments and treatments should reflect these. Our current approach is to apply generalized pathways and treatments, and this could be improved. Individuals can already be easily risk stratified into a 7% versus 46% likelihood of a syncope recurrence in 1 year, suggesting that future improvements might be on the horizon. Can the history be used in a more targeted fashion? Which specific patients would benefit from tilt testing or implantable loop recorders? Can recorders be developed that will detect blood pressure and other differences during syncope? And what about genomic and other biomarkers?

Grand challenge 5: Develop an individualized approach to most patients with syncope by 2020.

These goals although ambitious can be reached. Above all, the distress and needs of the patient must be remembered. There is a growing number of enthusiastic syncope investigators in fields ranging from physiology to health services delivery and at least 2 well-established international networks of syncope investigators that are already beginning to interact. With focus, funding, and synergy, a second golden age of syncope could mature in 2020.

Index

Note: Page numbers of article titles are in **boldface** type.

Cardiol Clin 31 (2013) 145–149
http://dx.doi.org/10.1016/S0733-8651(12)00133-6
0733-8651/13/$ – see front matter © 2013 Elsevier Inc. All rights reserved.

Moving?

Make sure your subscription moves with you!

To notify us of your new address, find your **Clinics Account Number** (located on your mailing label above your name), and contact customer service at:

Email: journalscustomerservice-usa@elsevier.com

800-654-2452 (subscribers in the U.S. & Canada)
314-447-8871 (subscribers outside of the U.S. & Canada)

Fax number: 314-447-8029

Elsevier Health Sciences Division
Subscription Customer Service
3251 Riverport Lane
Maryland Heights, MO 63043

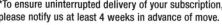
*To ensure uninterrupted delivery of your subscription, please notify us at least 4 weeks in advance of move.

ELSEVIER

Printed and bound by CPI Group (UK) Ltd, Croydon, CR0 4YY

03/10/2024

01040346-0014